*THE*

*Matthew Tree*

# THE MATTHEW TREE

BY H. T. WRIGHT

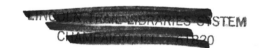

*PANTHEON BOOKS*

*A Division of Random House, New York*

*Library of Congress Cataloging in Publication Data*

Wright, H. T.

The Matthew Tree.

1. Euthanasia.  2. Stroke patients.  I. Title.

R726.W7      362.1'9'681      74–23689

ISBN 0–394–49592–6


H. T. Wright is a pseudonym.


Manufactured in the United States of America

FIRST EDITION

*With apologies to those I've embroidered*

There used to be a poor old woman who had only two chickens, one sick and the other healthy. Early one Friday morning she killed the healthy chicken to make soup for the sick one.

ANONYMOUS

# PART I

"Why," he had said. "Why?"

No mistake, we had both heard it.

Mother had been startled into dropping a couple of green stitches. I'd stared at my pencil independently adding an "A" in the last square of 38 Across. After weeks of comatose silence, "Why?"

Hardly expecting him to pull out of the in-between land, we had all wondered at Dad's first word. And here we were years later; again, plaintively, no longer expecting any answer, "Why?" Then he slipped back into his private world while Mother smoothed the pillows, tugged at the collar of his pajamas till no wrinkle dared lump behind his neck, asked, "What is it, dear? What is it? What can I do for you?" and sighed back into her chair when no response could come. I slumped back too, exhausted. The intricate guard over thousands of days and nights began to crumple, and scenes shoved at one another, vying for attention.

# PART II

# ONE

"Is THIS an emergency, Mrs. Wright?"

Lacking the certainty of severe or gory distress, I am intimidated by Dr. Mooney's brusque, practiced telephone tone. Unenviable decision: Am I wasting his time, or does my problem outshine all the others in his waiting room? Is it sufficiently startling that Dad's inner apparatus—polite but firm—had hurled into a waiting basin his baked haddock and noodles-with-cheese dinner, and that he had been apologetically, languidly, absolutely mute ever since? Or is such an upheaval not worthy of costly professional priority? How comforting to learn I've judged correctly! We are rewarded with an ambulance ride, bumpy, casual, and in no apparent hurry.

We begin the vigil, Mother and I—when she can, my sister, too—finding hospital routine by turns compassionate and efficient or indolent, pettishly performed by the underpaid. "Aides," an experienced visitor tells us, "are like yellow pencils. Use 'em for a while and then throw 'em away." Dad used to say that the best luck a person could have is, when his time comes, to go quickly. The thought must pierce his coma because he refuses all nourishment and keeps pulling out the intravenous. They finally reinsert it into the arm that still can move, tying him helpless, forcing him to live. My sister and I reassure one another that he is a good man, an exceptional man, he'd earn his wish not to become a burden.

A solemn Protestant minister makes his rounds; we recognize him from other sojourns in this hospital. His hair is all white now, but he's still so erectly handsome, he would make an admirable stand-in should Spencer Tracy again play a man-of-the-cloth. As in the past, he asks first whether we would like him to stop by. When we explain that we're not of his faith, he answers kindly that this makes no difference to him or to God. He comes in every day, takes Dad's hand, and with a soft, "Let us pray," bends his head in silence. I wonder—when the possibility of a recovery is remote—just what it is he's praying for.

Mother's needles gobble up hank after hank after hank of wool. I'm armed with spiral-bound crossword puzzles edited by Margaret Farrar, placemats and napkins stenciled for cross-stitch roses and back-stitch stems, and *147 Ways to Play Solitaire* in paperback. I master the noiseless shuffle. Phoning the family with lack-of-progress bulletins gets me out of the room periodically; these conversations at times realign a perspective, but then lose it in widening ripples of repetition. I come to depend upon the vagaries of the Bell System as an outlet for righteous complaints, and an occasional cliffhanger: Will they mail me my lost dime?

Dad is there five weeks when the woman puttering over her husband in the next room says, "My George had a stroke too, it will be seventeen months and one week next Thursday." A curious way of counting, more for measuring babies and the newly married. We listen to an endless retelling of George's condition and her daily worries, and murmur, "How dreadful, how terribly unfortunate."

The nurse apologizes for trying to force Dad to sip through a straw. She slides her hand behind the pillow to cradle his head securely. She tickles his nose to rouse him, calls his name and coaxes repeatedly, wets his lips with a drop of eggnog, prods and pushes at his cheeks till her fingermarks show. She gives up, saying, "This is for the birds," and silently I cheer him on toward what I still hope will be rapid, painless self-destruction.

It might be a Tuesday that his prosperous brother-in-law comes to visit and, for what unimaginable reason, lifts the covers—perhaps to see what Dad's lower parts look like, since no one had ever seen him barelegged even on the beach. Or maybe to check if his bunions are in as bad shape as the rest of him. He kicks at Uncle Harry's hand, frightening the poor man into dropping the blankets and fleeing the hospital.

Dad has made his first contrived movement.

Recovery commences.

## TWO

LIFE WAS SIMPLER all those years before the second car. Someone else did the driving, or our kids walked to school when it rained. In my bicycle basket there was no radio preoccupied with the ironies of war "casualties," with murders and suicides and how many little children died in senseless fires. Until the license and the old Olds stamp me Available.

I stop at a gas station where an attendant applies young muscles to the onetime-automated canvas top. As I adjust visor mirror and sunglasses, he breathes a low whistle of appreciation at my convertible. Off I go this lovely spring day, to investigate a succession of nursing homes.

Converted country mansions with wide verandas and airy rooms, big brick squares in the city, sparse, sleekly modern, antiseptic, dingy, homey, well-staffed or indifferent, they share the smell of Lysol, urine, and kitchen steam. We settle on one with an impressive building fund, a socially prominent board of directors, and endowments modestly named in brass in the lobby. Dad is provided with a different plastic name bracelet, and he gets two rolls of personalized tapes at no extra charge. Mother sews them on dozens of pajamas, two of her prized afghans. Like labeling the kids' clothes for camp.

Dad gets to know his left hand, his speech slowly returns though he interposes letters and mixes up words. His personality changes. He's sweet and mild as always with us, gets violently angry at times with Mother. She's dazed at first, then solidly positions herself: "He has to let it out at someone." None of us can remember exactly how his voice sounded last December.

We meet a massive master sergeant returned from her two-week stint in the Marine Reserves: the head nurse back from vacation. She is adamant. Dad needs the sociability of others and must therefore eat his meals from his wheelchair in the dining room. He is nauseated at the table with three other gentlemen who don't know the difference between sliced peaches and buttered noodles. I have a long conversation with the director, explaining that Dad's mind is altogether clear, that he is not to be branded Institutionalized, that he's a different kind of person. "He'll learn," I am told. "They all do." We're so many worlds apart in philosophies and attitudes and standards, I give up trying to communicate with this new authority, and win my way only by suggesting we'll find another place.

His trays are then brought into his room, and he discovers that an impossible soft-boiled egg is conquerable when slipped into cereal. He steadies his little finger against the side of the cup and can soon pour milk into his coffee and coffee into himself without losing any. We are reminded that when some guest at home refused a second Seagrams V.O., Dad never spilled a drop pouring it back into the bottle.

Dad's roommate here is about the same age, finicky in his unhappiness, a few months closer to mobility. Proud of his progress, Mr. Samuels tries to get ready for bed by himself one evening, twists blankets and night clothes into a widening knot, and meekly rings for help. The orderly who answers is maddened by the tangle, and, shoving at the old man, knocks him to the floor. Dad shakes at the bedrail and wildly raises his fist at the attendant: You're some hero—hitting a sick old man! *"You've got two hands!"* Mr. Samuels looks over the edge of the bed at Dad, tears sliding onto the floor.

We decide not to tell his daughters when they come.

I seek out the therapist one day, asking when exercises should begin. He is new there and, surprised he hasn't heard of Dad, comes to see him in his room. A couple of days later he advises me that physiotherapy should have begun months ago, before rigidity could have done so much harm. He works with Dad three times a week. He looks the other way as he tells me, "I'm terribly sorry, but to be honest with you, it's too late for appreciable results. I'm afraid that the most I can offer him now is psychological help."

Repeating this to the director—questioning her judgment and abilities—I am embroiled in deadly verbiage, and quickly outwitted by her facility with administrative loops and tangents. Later I realize that I was defeated from the very beginning of our argument, because only one of us really cared about my father.

I wonder what the rules are in such situations. Is this the only way to learn them? I shove the whole noxious bit into one of the compartments to be healed by time, and hope to be more alert in the future to troubles that are showered on the defenseless. I wish someone else— someone more capable—were in charge of this mess.

We move on to another convalescent home.

This place boasts an activities/social room, and patients are steered, wheeled, toted in for entertainment. One week a priest comes with a choir of children from the nearby parochial school; the next, a rabbi appears in his robes to do his thing. I offer to play the piano, and brush up on hymns and old ethnic tunes. We have community singing too, and soon the old people are arriving way ahead of time for the Wednesday treat.

Bolder in our programing, we ask for requests. A dotty little woman always responds immediately—in fact we can't ever stop her from asking for "Daisy, Daisy." We learn from a nurse that she hums it incessantly, often leading her private band far into the night.

They aren't the most discerning of audiences, but they are appreciative. At least they don't burn holes in the seats; hardly ever do they pee in the aisles.

One Wednesday during our "Favorites Time" an orderly taps me on the shoulder, whispering that his charge is new here and very shy. Although she's not an old woman, she's badly affected by Parkinson's disease. When we urge her, she hesitantly makes her request and I feel my way around the old show piece. It's not a familiar song for most of the folks, so there's general noise and disorder. But suddenly a clear, sweet soprano voice rises—amazingly unfaltering for one so wasted—hushing everyone to shocked attention: "Others find peace of mind in pretending—couldn't you, couldn't I, couldn't we . . . make believe . . . " She finishes to generous applause and even one feeble bravo, and I see that several nurses are digging in their pockets for Kleenex, just as I am.

A minor miracle sets to work in this place, and in a few months Dad is actually recuperating. Although his whole right side is paralyzed and he can't stand up by himself, he's strong enough now to sit in a chair.

"Do you think it's possible to bring Dad back to live with us?" First I ask fat Dr. Mooney, then a couple of talented nurses.

Opinions concur: "There's no medical reason why not, but it won't be easy. Do you think you can manage?"

Davy Crockett materializes before me, purposefully leading a file of Vikings around King Arthur's table of knights. Waggling a finger in proper form, I truck on ahead, leading Davy. Many, many are the shapes of Adventure.

My husband and I rearrange our house, calling on the kids' friends to help shove furniture around, wondering what providence had suggested we buy this home with two bedrooms on the first floor. I become acquainted with the soaring surgical supply industry. While I compare rental prices, a little boy investigates all the sample mechanisms; to him these showrooms are amusement parks with free rides. We get a hospital bed, wheelchair, and—trying not to dwell on the indignity—a portable adult-sized potty. We borrow sandbags from the fire department to keep Dad's legs straight in bed.

Next we tackle the help situation, uncomfortably aware of how much we'll be relying on the someone we hire. Always a modest man, painfully independent, Dad can't now tolerate the idea of anyone but Mother or a nurse tending to his more personal needs. I admit to myself that I'd dread having to do any of it anyhow.

We contract to import a middle-aged woman who, the employment man promises me, is very strong and thoroughly trained as a practical nurse. I drive to New York to pick her up. When we return home, I phone my sister: "Remember all those times I've said to you, 'Take it easy, don't worry'? Well, as of now, don't take it easy. I think we should all worry."

We take a big gulp, hope we can swallow all we've chewed, and bring Dad home.

Mother and the nurse don't like each other from the moment they're introduced. "I am on a very special diet," she informs us, as she uses a bar of butter to fry eggs for her lunch, spackling grease over the wall of our fresh new kitchen. Mornings, she sleeps so soundly that Mother has trouble waking her. She wears layer upon layer of clothes even on the warmest days. She saves old newspapers and used plastic bags under her bed. She wrings her hands a lot as she watches Mother tending to Dad.

She decides it's terrible that Dad hasn't had a bath in all these months. She undresses him, scoops him up in her arms, plunges him into the bathtub. Dad can't swim, but he gets a sensational ducking. Now it's my turn to pace the hall, wringing my hands, listening to the wild yells from the bathroom. How she ever gets him out of there and back into bed I am grateful not to witness. Dad is exhausted, sleeps for hours; our Nurse is tremendously proud of her Nursing.

Demoting our helper professionally, I spend a day answering Housekeeper Wanted ads in the paper and talking at great length on the phone. I deliver her into the arms of a desperate new employer with several small children on a farm out in Jersey. On the way home, alternately congratulating myself and writhing with guilt, I know that I will look back at this from the future and laugh. But sometimes it's rough to wait till I can look back and laugh.

## THREE

WE'RE FORTUNATE to replace our nurse with an aide from the local hospital. Pat drives her own car and is conscientious, so we don't mind too much when she monopolizes conversations at the dinner table or gradually intrudes in other family matters. We specifically ignore the sneaky doubt that she might drink a little. She's kind to Dad and he fares well.

We choose a mild fall day, bundle him up, and maneuver him into the car for a ride, pillows and safety belts propping him up in the front seat. He marvels at the autumn trees, at the people in the streets, at every store front and traffic light. Heady with success, we plan an excursion to visit our older daughter Susan, who is living in a garage apartment across the river. Pat is an acrobatic gem, getting Dad in and out of the car, into the wheelchair. He manipulates his wheels cautiously through the narrow dark hallway, peering into tiny rooms, eyes wide at the way two pretty, ever-so-slightly-hip college girls are managing their lives. We have a festive homemade chocolate mousse, and hug one another in delight.

Twice a week a physiotherapist comes to our house. He's friendly and jolly, tells us often how bad his back is and how much money he's making under Medicare. With slings, canes, and his own encouraging arms he manages to "walk" Dad across the room. He's there when two insurance men arrive to investigate the claim they've been paying. They're unctuous, solicitous, furious. They're the ones who'd persuaded Dad to buy this exceptional policy just one year and two days before he took ill. As he slowly recognizes them, Dad grins at Mother and points a shaky index finger skyward, apologetically reminding the heavens how the soul can be gratified triumphing over a million-dollar corporation like Continental Casualty. The therapist chuckles his way down the front walk, gleeful as he leaps into his silver Cadillac.

Novelty gives way to routine.

Dad laboriously grows a mite stronger, and we look for ways of occupying his time. When the kids are home for a holiday weekend we sprawl over the living room floor, coaxing the change we've saved for years out of the neck of a two-gallon cider jug, pouring it into pots, jars, mixing bowls. We bring the bathroom scale: thirty-nine and a half pounds of money, net. Dad spends afternoons in his wheelchair at the dining table with a dozen quart-sized ice cream containers, first sorting the coins, then patiently peering through a little magnifying glass at both sides of each one, searching for important dates or imperfections. After checking with interminable lists in a numismatic manual, he presents us with a half-pint of hopefuls, which I promise to take for a professional collector's appraisal.

"If you bring me some pill bottles, I think I can manage the rest," he suggests. So we scour the medicine chests and junk drawers, though none of us can guess what he wants with them. We watch as he selects four different sizes to fit quarters, nickles, pennies, dimes, then carefully counts out a sample pile of each. With the tip of his finger he measures the height of a stack of un-distinguished coins. He folds the bottom of a money wrapper, fills a pill bottle with coins, empties it into the paper cylinder, and tucks the top together neatly. My husband and I try it that night using only one hand and ask one another, How the hell does he do it?

He's proud of his rolled-up $893.50, miserable be-cause he has to watch me carry the heavy carton out to the car myself. I bring it to the bank, discover I should have noted our account number on the wrappers along with the name and address. A teller hands me a pen, insists that I write 131-206814 on each roll. When I tell Dad, he is incensed, shaking his head for days over petty officialdom.

Pat doesn't show up one Friday. She answers the phone in a slurred voice when we call. We tell her to feel better, and I silently add, please, please sober up.

Mother assures me that everything will be all right for the afternoon, and I go to the market, annoyed when I unerringly pick the slow checkout line. While I'm gone, Mother tries to help Dad up after his nap, but they don't quite manage to slide him off the edge of the bed into the chair. He slumps onto the floor like a Raggedy Andy, his "bad" side crumpled beneath him, one leg hooked under the bed. Mother tries and tries to budge him, till she has to sit down quietly and reach for her nitroglycerin tablets.

It seems hours that they stay this way, taking turns at comforting one another, till the back bell rings and our laundry man opens the door with his customary, "Hi there, anybody home?" Knowing there should be, he finds his way through the house until Mother calls.

He awkwardly tugs and pulls at Dad, finally bounces him face down on the bed and turns him over politely. He waits till I come home and we sit in the bedroom with tea and cookies, watching the late fall sun begin to set.

I call Pat to make sure she can come in the next day, and then post the police station number in big print on the telephone extensions.

*       *       *

It's nearly Christmas time. Our daughter Alicia impulsively promises a cookie house for the senior class "hospital project," and the whole family gets involved. We overrule Mother who wants to bake dozens and dozens of cookies, and buy them instead, along with food coloring and huge amounts of confectioners' sugar. Dad is appointed direction-master, Mother is in charge of mixing enormous batches of icing. Late in the afternoon we start on the cardboard base. Dad wheels round and round the kitchen, excitedly overseeing every process, holding the instructions in his lap, pointing a finger of advice. We make mistakes along the way, but fortunately cover them with icing. We are so absorbed every day after school, all other kitchen business is suspended for the rest of the week. We agree at last that this is indeed an unparalleled cookie house, and take turns snapping the Polaroid from every angle.

Early Saturday when Alicia's friend comes to help her deliver the precious work, I watch from the door as she gingerly carries it to the car—and slips just as she reaches the curb, tumbling onto a snowbank mid a disaster of cookies. I see Freddy slowly help her to her feet, overhear him, nervous, doomed, say, "It was the logical thing, Lish. It had to happen." She is too stunned to do anything but stare at him. I have to walk around the room twice before I dare to tell Dad and Mother.

Planting flowers in front of the house in the spring, I find a few little petrified cinnamon candies, which I turn into the soil. They must be of horticultural value because that year we have exceptional, hardy, lovely pansies.

Once I stood on a corner carrying a big flat board with a plaster-of-Paris relief map of India for—could it be fifth grade?—geography class. My father had helped me patiently, meticulously, with it. As I waited to be crossed, a sudden gust of wind attacked the oaktag and felled my prized Himalaya chain, powdering it into the Indian Ocean. Lish and I talk about it, trying to weigh psychological effect, sharing a vulnerability to the elements.

＊　＊　＊

Pat appears regularly, though suspiciously wobbly on occasion. We are so thankful for her help that we include a bottle of Scotch in her holiday gifts.

＊　＊　＊

Establishing a balance of attention between husband and children, parents, and the outside world threatens to be overwhelming. The freeness of our private humor, the easiness of our special banter is no longer available to my husband and me. Our sex life has been dealt a serious blow. The sweetest part of our time together depends on a rarefied, deliciously personal environ that suffers when "outsiders" are around for too long a while. We are glad the children are grown; it would be terribly difficult for them and for us to deal with them if they were younger and needed more of us.

I berate myself for not having had a full-time job of even mediocre import, which could take precedence over these present concerns. I envy my sister the financial need that requires her to work every day, and the insulating miles between her home and mine. I force myself to examine all the resentments, then squelch them one by one into the certainty that my conscience wouldn't allow me to do any less than I am doing. If I've cried myself out under a long hot shower, beating on the tiles in frustration, my husband kisses me gently and says, "You can't help doing what you're doing. That's the way you're stuffed."

## FOUR

STROKE TWO. Aha, we say. This is how you learn the ropes.

Accomplished now, we declare an emergency and Dr. Mooney comes immediately. We call the local police for an ambulance, and they arrive almost as the phone is put back on the hook. Two tall young cops, short-haired and serious, assure Dad that everything will be all right, "Don't you worry, Sir." When they ask me to please let them know if there's anything else they can do, I swear to argue down anyone who ever says "pig."

Mother rides in the ambulance, smoothing out the lines of Dad's forehead, trying to be reassuring as he stares at her wonderingly, silently, then closes his eyes into deeper unawareness. I follow in the car through red lights and traffic. At the hospital the doctor warns, "We don't have much to work with this time." I remind him that Dad wouldn't want him to knock himself out look-ing for much to work with, and neither do we. He nods and leans over confidentially: "We won't do anything heroic, but we must do the minimum."

And we do what we did last year.

Again Dad is unconscious for six weeks. Mother insists on visiting every day; we neither blame her nor find any other plausible transportation, so I chauffer again.

Sometimes it isn't really better second time around.

As we sit in his room, watching him hardly live, tenaciously unresponsive to the whimsical demands of society, I decide that someone must help ease him out of this minimum existence. Painlessly, quickly, peacefully, and with dignity, I must help him. He can't swallow, so pills are out. All usual means to the end are unapplicable here in this semiprivate room next to the nursing station. I try to recall detective stories but my mind rejects such reference if I force it to plan. I am biologically naïve, not detail-oriented. I have an inhibited imagination, a rotten memory, a terrible time lying. I have seen *The Maltese Falcon* four times in the past twenty-odd years and I still can't completely understand the plot. I wish I didn't like my father; I assume it's a simpler business to contemplate when prompted, spontaneously, by hate.

"To a better year," my husband and I clink glasses in front of the fireplace with two dearly close friends. We stare into the flames, each mesmerized. This is the first time the chant forms inside my head, to the beat of an old football cheer: "Let . . . Dad . . . die . . . now . . . Make it now, Make it now."

Next morning I type seven times:

MY DEAREST HUSBAND, MY DEAREST CHILDREN:

IF EVER I AM IN A CONDITION SIMILAR TO MY FATHER'S, PLEASE GET A FAST AND FINAL HAPPY PILL, OR SHOT, FROM A RELIABLE SOURCE, AND MAKE CERTAIN I ABSORB IT. THEN, IF YOU CARE TO, GO TO A MOVIE.

MANY THANKS AND MUCH LOVE,

H.T.W., JANUARY 1966

I fold the copies—dotted with Chanel No. 5—among nightgowns, pocketbooks, papers, and sewing stuff, in alternate drawers of my dresser and desk.

Winter drags into spring.

In the hospital corridor I meet Dr. Mooney, who shakes his head over this enigma: "He shouldn't have been able to pull out of this one, it was a beaut. I guess his time just isn't up yet."

As I'm reporting to uncles and aunts thirsting for details, a gold inlay comes flying out of my mouth, clattering to the floor of a favorite phonebooth. Shocking, to find that I welcome the respite at the dentist's! "You must be clenching your teeth too hard," he warns.

Dad takes to hiding his "bad" arm, objects furiously when the nurse overrules: he must keep it on a pillow on top of the blankets. He regards it as an alien, hateful thing, pushes and throws it about with a venomous snarl. The hospital makes noises about needing the bed for something more urgent, so we begin the convalescent home search once more for Dad, who has proceeded from bony to skinny to frail to fragile. In every respect he is less able, except for his mind which, when consciousness returns at all, surfaces to attention with the old unanswerable: "Why?"

Although we maintain the when-you're-well-enough-to-come-home attitude for both Dad and Mother, we decide on pragmatism: Inconceivable, but this *could* go on for a year or more; we'd best make some changes. Having moved several times before for various reasons— a roomier house, easier commuting, better school system—here's a valid one too, especially since the kids are away at college and will probably never live full-time with us again. Our role in the suburbs has come to an end.

We sell our house, and I miss my father acutely. He

was always a mainstay of calm, packing and unpacking with rhythmic efficiency, never a broken dish or smudge of newsprint on his white shirt. Once Dad is installed in the mercifully adequate Riverview Nursing Home, we find an apartment nearby, and arrange more compactly the necessities of everyday life. Changing surroundings is always refreshing, but this time the satisfying feeling of adapting to a new circumstance is in hourly jeopardy if we dare look beneath the surface of our decision. Much welcome busywork is to be done, like lining the shelves, stuffing books about, agreeing on just the right wall and height for pictures. And doing the laundry.

There is a nosy breed of women who find curious outlet in inspecting other people's wash. I could have made a host of friends if I'd followed through with intimate details: No, I don't work for a bachelor, I like to dress this way and all these pajamas are for my father who's ill; Yes, we iron them all; No, we don't have sleep-in help; No, these oversized bibs are not for my baby; Yes, they're for my father because he can't always eat neatly and drools a lot without feeling it. Comparing illness woes can tie fast social bonds. I think I must have an operation, though, in order to compete in a loftier league.

Soon someone steals a big deep-pink bath rug from the dryer; another low person exchanges our shiny new shopping cart for one that's scratched and squeaky. Even so, the chore could be much less attractive—if I had to rub all these pajamas on the stones of a nearby brook, or carry water up a hill from a not-nearby well, or stand on slatted boards in a dark cellar, scrubbing stains on a washboard set deep in a galvanized tub.

Impatient with waiting for the elevator, and with the two-whooshes-to-every-floor as it throbs down to the basement, I devise a game. Before I leave at the basement level, I press the button for the highest floor, then again for "B." I run into the laundry room, grab my clothes out of the washer, throw them into the dryer. If I win, I can fly into the elevator just as it reaches the basement again. This works only if (a) I have just one washer full of laundry; (b) there is an empty dryer waiting; (c) GE responds to my first quarter without hesitation; (d) no callous person on an intermittent floor wants to go up or down.

We draw a layout of the apartment for Dad, revising our sketch every time we shuffle the furniture. We make a map to show where we are in relation to the nursing home, the river, the highway, landmark skyscrapers he might remember.

He is in a semiprivate room for a few months with a succession of roommates who, with better luck than he, go home healed, expire quietly during the night, or, ensconced in senility, make a mockery of living.

Again I have a definitive chat with a supervisor, this time a sympathetic, experienced nurse. She's skeptical at the notion that Dad is *different,* but imaginative enough to consider a change in accommodations. When there's an opening, she suggests a private room, pointing out that since it faces the tiny courtyard, it's not too bright; over the utility room, it's likely to be warm and possibly noisy. We can have it for the same price. Mother declares that privacy is urgent; Dad is pleased with the choice. Bargains like this are not easy to unearth.

Opposite his bed we hang a moon-lit Florida seascape, a modest oil offered to the folks many years back by a talented young friend, and Dad is weepy when he looks at it. We bring a TV from home, a little white electric clock, an unbreakable candy jar of mock Delft, a small wooden cube with baby pictures of his grandchildren framed on each side, "Chip Off The Old Block" lettered in gold on the top. Mother adds a couple of pots of philodendron, a geranium balanced precariously on the narrow window sill, a vase of unlikely plastic roses. We prop up speedy recovery cards wherever we find a flat surface, and then pile them on the TV stand where Dad can easily see the growing number of get-well wishes. I drive Mother over at two, pick her up at six, spend varying amounts of time with them in-between. Several relatives visit regularly on Sunday afternoons, and with typical punctuality and consistency make those particular hours ritual.

A Saturday in the summer, with an okay from the head nurse and a lot of help from three aides, my husband and I take Dad out for a drive along the river. He's delighted for the first twenty minutes or so, but becomes anxious with the strain of trying to stay upright in the front seat. We shorten our route, decide not to point out our apartment (where, when he recovers, he will come back and live with mother and us), and return to the nursing home. We realize that he is fearful of his occasional incontinence, nervous that he might have an "accident" on the way. For weeks later he tells us, carefully etching each word, "Thank you. I thank you very much. I'm sorry. No more. I can't do it. No good."

He is reminded of the other drives we took, when he was at home with us in-between strokes. Though his speech is severely damaged, we can understand that those three months hover persistently—maybe exclusively—in spite of the seventy-nine active years that preceded them.

## FIVE

HAS HE SKILLFULLY shunted aside his earliest years? Or have they been eradicated as completely as his birthplace—a small farm in the middle of Europe? So many times had his homeland been gobbled up by larger countries, then spit back to stronger powers, that his countrymen themselves must have been confused about their boundaries, if not their allegiance.

When my sister and I were children, we'd ask Dad to tell us, again and again, of the time he was chased by hungry wolves on his way home from the village. He'd had to stop to inspect a limping wagon wheel, jumping back onto the seat to quiet his horse when the baying pack suddenly appeared. He'd tied the reins around a small tree and lit a firebrand for protection while he chopped at bits of ice crusted on the rim. Then he'd leapt back into the wagon and raced to the security of his yard, the wolves close on his back.

"How'd you know to start a fire? Did you always carry matches?" we would ask, conjuring up ferocious beasts that very moment slaloming down our own block, gracefully skirting the lamp posts. "If you were only nine or ten, how'd you know just what to do?"

"I *had* to know. We all had to know." My father's strength has always been a meld of disciplined intuition and practice.

He used to be surprised, but pleased, that we never tired of hearing the story, and he always told it the same way. The temperature never dropped, the wolves didn't multiply, the miles to safety didn't increase, and he was no more or no less frightened.

Do those same creatures ever lust across his night-time horizons now? I wonder.

And does he remember how he chose the exact moment to come to America? The first of ten children, Dad had entered this world with Responsibility grooved into each shoulder knob like a hollowed-out deformity. He arrived here, a teenager fluent in five languages, English not among them. He had to learn fast, make money fast; he had to help bring over the rest of his family—including his own parents, aged and ill, his youngest brother and sister, born after he'd left home. Did his genes conspire to form him stoic, plodding and imaginative, energetic and subdued? Are they the tiny culprits who commandeered duty and family to head his personal agenda? Or did Responsibility shape him . . . and as a result, he needed it as much as it needed him?

Not so unique for the sensitive among those first-born young immigrants of the early 1900s, he was to spend the next half-century fighting down the label Greenhorn.

Through American-born cousins, he met a mutual relative—a pretty young woman with a turned-up nose and shy, soft voice, who always walked as tall and as proud as she could. Born and raised on a demure farm in South Jersey, she was a newcomer to the city, exploring the complicated wonders of an outlandish book-keeping machine on the exciting seventh floor of the world's largest department store.

To approach this American girl in marriage was daring. He accomplished the deed by formally asking of her mother: "It's a long while since I've called anyone 'Mother.' May I call you that?" The reply was immediate: "I would be honored, and I know my daughter is too."

For all the years they were married, he was to shield his bride—as her father and brothers had earlier done—from such unsavories as mortgage payments, naughty politics, or taking out the garbage. (Perhaps the shieldee suffers more than the shielder: Mother's the one who has been racked by the insidious ploys of tension.)

I grew up taking for granted that everybody's family also lived serenely, quietly. Only when I was old enough to visit away from home for a few days at a time did I realize that ours was the unusual household—governed by a marriage free of bickering, nastiness, and malignant reprisals.

Just once—I was perhaps seven—can I recall knowing that there was a strain between my parents, but no voice was raised, no hint of recrimination localized it. For several hours the silence in the house just felt different. Then my mother came slinking down the stairs, decked out in long beads and something chiffon, scarves misting her face and head. She struck a Theda Bara pose in our tiny living room and executed a dance of her own seven veils for Dad, who leaned his elbow on the radiator and chuckled appreciatively, "Very nice. That's really lovely." My sister and I rolled onto the floor, screaming for more.

"Shhh, not so loud," said Mother, in and out of character. "What will the neighbors say?"

Just once do I remember Dad punishing us . . . does he? He hit my sister across the behind with his belt because she could spell "alpha" and she could spell "bet," but she couldn't spell "alphabet." Watching, I wailed as loud as she did; that spanking sufficed for both of us. So I grew up a little afraid of my father, but not questioning my love for him or convinced that a bit of judicious inhibition is altogether negative.

＊   ＊   ＊

Does he recall when my turn came to revolt against his authority? I struck out not against my father's influence —not against him as a person—but rather for the right to choose my own kind of life. Which he was ready to relinquish, suspecting that my way wouldn't differ so greatly from his. I fought with what I considered his limitations, realizing in later years that they were self-imposed and, like his prejudices and his relentless self-control, necessary for survival. I battled, too, with the Dragon of the Syndrome of Guilt, which my parents had unwittingly nourished; luckily no adherence to organized religion compounded that struggle. To my parents, guilt has more concrete ramifications, the word of Freud never having interfered with their tender psyches. Rigid but fair, they have always considered what people do as right or wrong; good acts proffer peace of mind; bad ones, guilt and shame. Not a simplistic approach, if one continually adds to and revises his list of standard deeds, and keeps his mouth shut over deep-down, honestly obnoxious thoughts.

Where, for instance, has Dad tucked away the scene in our living room, when I told my parents that I wanted to marry the guy who had just returned from hitchhiking cross-country, the one who hated wearing a tie, who had an unmatchable sense of humor and no job?

Dad and Mother had sat close together on the couch, holding hands, while I fidgeted on the piano bench, looking out the window and being incoherent.

"Are you sure this is what you want?" they hammered away at that toughest of questions. No need, really, to ruminate over faith and trust and the infinite meanings of love. When I finally was able to gulp, "I think so," they were instantly in accord: "Then go ahead, and be very happy." Whereupon Mother began planning a menu for the wedding, and this skinny rebel became the most desirable son-in-law in the world.

Describing to my father's father my catch of a fiancé, I chose to ignore the wardrobe and plug the sense of humor.

"Sensayuma?" Grandpa couldn't understand.

"That's right, he's got a great sense of humor. You have one, too, Grandpa. You like to laugh . . . you always laugh, like when you see people fall down."

Puzzled, Grandpa was probably thinking how nice if I were to marry a doctor. He looked a lot like a worried George Bernard Shaw. "Sensayuma means he likes it when other people hurt themselves?"

Long pause.

"No, not exactly. Don't worry—wait till you meet him. I know you'll like him."

"You like him?"

"Yes. I like him very much."

"I also like him. Sensayuma too."

＊　　＊　　＊

Why doesn't Dad recall the year before he took ill for the first time, the year he finally retired from eight hours a day tending bar in his own tavern, the swift year in the suburbs? He and Mother had been like a newly married couple in the tiny garden apartment crammed with forty-eight years of accumulated homemaking. The move from the city was an exciting challenge for them. There were new neighbors, shyly approached and conquered; the baby next door who learned as we all had that Mother's cinnamon pinwheels were to be devoured by unrolling them and licking the crumbs from a pudgy hand.

For Mother—primarily involved with housekeeping all her life—the change was merely of environ. Dad found the transition more difficult, so the rest of us organized a few creative thinking sessions for ways to occupy his time. I asked for ideas of part-time or volunteer work from a sociologist friend. When he learned that Dad was seventy-nine, he looked at me peculiarly and said, "You ask me for suggestions about a *job?*" Does geriatrics refer to age or capability or attitude? I wonder.

On his own, Dad potted about in the garage, subdued a jungle of cellar disarray, catalogued record albums. He sorted blue and green and plaid stamps, wrinkled and jammed in a shoe box, and neatly pasted them into redemption books. He supervised renovation of our kitchen, reckoning with the fat plumber who got stuck behind the refrigerator trying to connect an automatic ice cube dispenser. And he did the marketing, because he still drove, though I handed over the car keys with no small worry.

A friend in the movie business thoughtfully supplied a few reels of used 16mm. prints, which Dad was to test for quality of viewing. He rigged up a stand in the basement, taught himself to use the projector, crayoned scratches on the film, spliced and rewound endlessly. The rate of five dollars per reel was embarrassing, but he showed no hesitation: here was a job to be done. He wore a thick sweater as the weather turned cool, resented the time wasted on lunch, and kept a pace that threatened a hernia for my husband who lugged the heavy reels back and forth from the city.

When September came we pushed Adult Education brochures at them, and though protesting and reticent, they were both intrigued. Carefully scrubbed—Mother in a new blue and green print, Dad in a striped bow tie —they were waiting under a wide maple tree when I pulled up to drive them to the local high school for enrollment. "Aren't you a little late?" they asked. I signed up for Cybernetics, since it was given at the same hours, and nighttime chauffeuring could be dismissed easily in the light of "I'm going too." Mother favored Advanced Dressmaking. She rejected Gourmet Cooking after seeing a list of ingredients in recipes that would be tackled over the term, setting forever forth for her own perennially disgestible pot roast and stuffed cabbage.

We still have the shade pulls, Christmas ornaments, and paperweights of stained glass that Dad fashioned, peering over his bifocals at surprisingly bold color patterns; the notched cutting boards lovingly sanded for his granddaughters' future choppings. Toward the end of the first term a little party was held at the home of one of his classmates. Mother took time from her class to go too, and came away justly proud of Dad's revered spot among fellow students scores of years his junior.

They had made a sweet and remarkable adjustment to

retirement; it was all the more painful when, after Dad took ill, we had to disband the apartment because Mother couldn't keep it alone. We managed a sublease, packed, stored, sold, and gave away a household of memories.

# SIX

I$\text{T'S}$ SEVENTEEN MONTHS and one week since the first stroke, one hundred seventy-two days since the second. We settle into a holding pattern circling round the four-hour stint in the nursing home. White uniforms gradually separate into personalities who perform a gamut of duties for Dad's functioning. They dose him with supplements of supplements to vitamins to keep him healthy, antibiotics and shots to keep him from being sick. They clean him, shave him, superintend his plumbing. They tie him in the straight-backed armchair during the morning and again after midday rest. A couple of times a week they go through the motions of standing him up, but Dad realizes as well as we that it's only a gesture, and soon this little act is discontinued. They tell us that he often asks them "Why?" but they don't know what he means.

He receives lots of mail and visitors offering hard fruit candies, Black Belt Aftershave Lotion, a hopeful plaid robe which must be returned to Bloomingdale's. And plants in great variety, most of which Mother brings home with the admonition, "There's really not enough sun to grow it here." One wispy Jerusalem cherry tree is spirited away immediately, deposited on a corner table in our living room where the light will be just right. She fusses over it, turns it every day, till it prospers evenly and soon must be transplanted to a larger pot.

Mother's daily chores occupy her completely. She irons pajamas, cooks and bakes for my husband and me, makes pudding and soup for Dad. "He eats so little. At least if he takes what I bring, I know that he's getting that much nourishment." She trots the portions over along with clean pajamas, white socks, neatly bound bibs cut from old pink terry cloth towels, her knitting, two spoons, and a milk-glass dessert dish with a fluted rim double-wrapped in aluminum foil and rubber bands.

I drop her off at the curb and watch as she lugs her flowered vinyl shopping bag up the few front steps, pulls open the heavy double doors, turns, and waves me on. She smiles pleasantly at the receptionist, and continues up the stairs, leaning the shopping bag against her knee as she shoves at the massive iron gate set across the stairwell to keep the right ones in and the right ones out. She greets the nurses, makes her way down the hall. She flicks on the light switch at Dad's room, and with a cheerful, "Hello, darling, how are you today?" stashes items in closet and drawers, checks candy and Kleenex supply, pushes back the night table, turns on the TV.

Holding hands, they sit side by side looking at the Tube from two to three-thirty, as absorbed in the commercials as the soap operas. (Watching "The Secret Storm" with them one afternoon when the good guy is suffering a particularly luckless time, I say to Dad, "You think you've got troubles—look at him!" Dad turns toward me, raises his hand palm out for a moment, then lets it fall limply, in what has become a characteristic gesture of his resignation and despair. I am uneasy with my leaden attempt.)

Out in the hall the parade of patients forms. There's Emil, who knows little English, answering before you ask him how he is with a rapid-fire "Fine fine fine fine-finefinefine." His daughter is a teacher in a nearby school; she comes to visit him every other month, and after a few minutes they have violent quarrels. For several days afterwards he throws whatever he can manage at whoever enters his room. Probably better for uninitiated ears that he spills out his invective in his own Old World tongue.

There's Rosie, a crumpled-up, misshapen little thing with the awesome black eyes of a gypsy. She drones a steady "Bella Rosa" while reciting the rosary of her sweater buttons. And Mrs. Ames, tall, straight, and slim, fingering an unopened *New York Times* folded over the bar of her walker: each to his own security blanket. She has a deep, cultured voice, a charming manner, and never any visitors. For months she has insisted countless times a day—always with the air of a startling discovery —that her engagement ring and notebook have been stolen, that she truly wants a cigarette. (Why, oh *why* shouldn't she be allowed to smoke all she pleases, with cancer at age eighty-four? How much more can there be in store? How much more to preserve?)

And then there's the man who looks like Lon Chaney in the hunchback role, who cries all the time; the stout old fellow who, in the middle of the corridor im-mediately after dinner, methodically starts to remove his trousers; the inseparable duo, one woman a foot and a half shorter than her prim friend, both shuffling about in bobby socks and huge men's slippers; the lumpy lady who whimpers near the gate and punches any passerby on the arm. And the heavy-set, youngish-looking man who waits at the desk, asking about the schedule of the bus that's due here and has he missed it; the curly-headed black woman with a sweet smile and no legs; Johnson, tall on one side and terribly disfigured on the other, who assures everyone he's "just getting along"; deaf Mr. Foster, perky and mod in his tennis sneakers and red flannel shirt, incontinence staining his blue jeans.

Eagerly they grope their way along the handrails, progress painfully with walkers and canes, push one another ahead in wheelchairs. They wave and call to Dad from the doorway as they march on—half an hour early, some of them—to the highlight of their day: puréed dinner.

Dad's meals are brought in on trays. (He manages two by himself, but Mother insists on feeding him his dinner, zealous over every spoonful as with an underweight child.) I come back between five and six, and Mother and I lean against the wall outside his room while two attendants put him back to bed. He thanks them, invites them to have a candy as they roll up soiled bed linens and leave him fixed for the night. The room smells of rubbing alcohol and Johnson's Baby Powder.

Although before he took ill Dad always had an ardent interest in the affairs of the world, he refuses now to look at a magazine or paper. I scrape the inside of my head for topics and people to talk about, while Mother chats too and knits away on her current afghan. Then come her leaving rituals: cleaning his fingernails, measuring candies out into a shallow tin, checking on sandbags, blankets, and sheepskin mat, folding three Kleenexes around the edge of his collar to catch unfelt saliva, three more lined up on his chest. (We buy only colored tissues; he can't see white ones against the sheet.)

I crank the head of the bed up or down at his explicit direction, as Mother shimmies the nightstand back into place. Dad eyes it closely, reaches over to check the precise angle from which he can get a candy and the nighttime supply of Kleenex fluffing out of the box. Mother raises the bedrail, ties the bell, adjusts the clock till he says, "All right. Good."

"Good-night, dear, have a good night," Mother hopes, kissing him good-bye.

"Sleep well, Dad." I kiss his forehead, and he kisses the hand I've patted his with. We turn off the light switch outside his door, and wrench ourselves away from the sinewy hand he waves, the wistful kiss he blows in return.

"That's all right, I can carry it, it's not heavy," says Mother.

"I don't mind," and I take the shopping bag, now containing a plastic bag of laundry knotted at the top and stuffed deep inside where no one can peer at it. Did life really exist before plastic?

"At least he has no bedsores—his bed is immaculate," says Mother. I agree.

"They use up an awful lot of candy," says Mother, "but at least I know that they stop in to see how he is."

"That's true, I know."

"You know, in all the years I know him, never once has Dad said, 'I'm hungry,' or 'I'm thirsty.' Only that he might have a little something. Never did I hear him say he was hot or cold or tired. The most he would ever say is that it's chilly or it's warm out, or maybe he would lie down for a few minutes. He never rings the bell either."

"Yes, I know."

"Oh well," sighs Mother as we get into the car.

She's uncomplaining, indomitable, more active than she's been in years. She has glaucoma, a damaged heart, arthritis, gallstones, diverticulitis, varicose veins, a bad back, and a truculent bladder. She's cute. She's incredible. She pops a phenobarb three times a day and one or two Seconal to sleep.

      ✿    ✿    ✿

I drive down to the river in clear mid-November to walk through the deserted picnic area. Ours is a great city river—not skinny like the Seine, or jostled like the Thames, or murky like the Danube, or barren like the Moskva. Or sad and heroic like the Charles. This river, like a sweep of ocean, often makes me think of death, and of those dear in the past who—through my recurrent little-child view—look down from the skies but no longer see it. I contemplate its shores and my navel. I miss the blessed freedom of being responsible only to my husband, only for our two daughters. I hate this new paradoxical power over my parents: I dutifully bestow my favors by visiting, by clearing away a larger space for them in my cozy inner world, till their mounting obligation, like their need, is devastating to contemplate.

The reversal of our roles is being pushed too far, like a tasteless practical joke: On long summer days, when I was a kid, I'd loll after my mother, complaining that I had nothing to do. Nowadays my mother follows me about the house when she's in-between afghans and the cookies are cooling, asking, "What shall I do now?"

How does a nice girl like me, caught in a spot like this, go about breaking her mold and cracking up? If I could manage a small nervous breakdown, a dimension of excitement might be added. Is it enough for openers that I can barely force myself to get out of bed at noon? That when my husband leaves in the morning I stay there, pulling the covers over my head and wishing myself back to sleep? That I'm constantly on the prowl for a cold so I can stay home—but then have to cope with Mother, all concerned about my backache, trudging over to Riverview in a cab? That with me at all times is a gawdy oval pill box with a single Equanil left over from somebody else's 1963 trauma? How to creep out from under? Where to run away to? How to shuck a conscience?

I complain to the water, accuse the trees: "I am so bored I can't stand it. I think I'm going out of my mind."

I look at my watch, it's quarter to five. I move toward the car to go pick up Mother at the Riverview Nursing Home.

Activity, activity, that's the answer: keep busy and you'll keep out of trouble. I've done my time on volunteer brigades in the suburbs, chaired the cupcake division of three PTAs and one PTO. There's no Roosevelt, Stevenson, or Henry Wallace to inspire me to stuff and seal. A lot of liquor makes me conk out, so becoming an alcoholic is not promising. I'm too vain to succumb to the Solace of Chocolates, too stubborn to surrender myself to tranquilizing agents. I know the measure of my desperation when I start cleaning closets. Where I find a garment bag and a big box covered with the untorn part of a faded print blanket cover . . . Mother saves everything and uses it all. As though bound for overseas, the carton is tied with slip knots and half-hitches. It's full of Dad's clothes.

Tucked among the underwear are checkbook and bank statements, an old address book. Seeing that careful handwriting again is a jolt; now only on an extra special greeting card for the kids will he attempt a shaky, feathery, lefthanded "POP." We give away dress shirts, ties, and shoes; but Mother keeps an overcoat, hat, and winter robe, "just in case." It's four-and-a-half years later that she's able to admit they probably won't be needed any more.

## SEVEN

"HEL-LO, MR. DANIELSON. How are you today?" I stop down the hall to see one of Dad's former roommates. His daughter and son are there too; with the precision of persons who declare Tuesday's at 10 A.M. Shoelace Washing Time, Emily and Len appear for their weekly visit.

"How're things, Mr. Danielson?" I take his hand in an attempted shake. "How're you doing?"

"Look at that, Len. Poppa's trying to look up at her. I bet he thinks she's Anna. Remember his niece Anna?"

"Of course I remember Anna. Why shouldn't I remember Anna?" Len is quick to his own defense.

Mr. D. purses his lips, and daughter Emily bends close over him.

"Listen, Len. Len, did you hear him?"

"What? No, I didn't hear him. Did he say something?"

"It sounded like he said your name. What did you say, Poppa?"

Poppa looks around, flicks a nonexistent mosquito from his ear. He fumbles in his lap, through folds of his sweater and a bunched-up sheet securing him to the chair. He chuckles, frowns, leers at a thread.

"It's nice out today, but very warm, Mr. Danielson."

"Yes, it is warm out today, isn't it, Len? Poppa, did you hear that? It's warm out today."

"You're wearing a very nice sweater today, Mr. Danielson." I pat his concave chest. "I like this sweater."

"Watch Poppa, Len. He knows it's his sweater! He's feeling the edge of the binding. He's looking at a button. See that, Len?"

Mr. D. studiously places a crumb on the tray table before him, feels around for a forgotten tool.

Len is attentive: "What are you looking for there, Poppa?"

"Will this do, Mr. Danielson?" I hand over a spoon from the nightstand behind him. Mr. D. eyes it warily, takes it slowly by the handle. He runs his fingers over the table surface till he finds his crumb, peers at it suspiciously. He slow-motions hammering at the crumb with the spoon.

"Look, Len—Poppa thinks he's hammering something. Remember how he used to love to hammer things? . . . No, no, Poppa. Len, take the spoon from him. He mustn't bang like that."

"That's all right, it's okay for him to do that. What's the difference if he bangs? He likes to have something in his hands, don't you, Poppa?"

"But, Len, he'll put it in his mouth. He might choke on it, Len."

"We'll be here watching. It'll be all right. Won't it, Poppa?"

"I don't think so, Len." Worried, Emily looks at me for confirmation.

"Why don't you give him something to hammer with —maybe a little rubber mallet and some blocks? Then he could hammer all he wants," I suggest.

"Oh no, we couldn't do that. He'd probably break them." She moves to take away the spoon, which Poppa hangs onto in a knotted, arthritic grip.

I look around the double-occupancy room. Mr. D's current roommate, tied in his chair between the beds, his back curved till nose nears knees, incessantly staccatoes on the arm of his protective cage, irrevocably lost to the outer world. Other than this partner, sparse hospital furniture, and two flower pots on the window sills behind the curtains, Mr. D. has nothing in this room to look at, nothing in this world to do. I panic at the thought. "But he wants to do something with his hands —why not give him something harmless to occupy them with?"

His daughter takes the spoon, and Mr. Danielson feels about for a screwdriver, or pliers, perhaps. "We can't give him children's things to play with—that's degrading," she shudders.

"But if he hammers with a spoon, why not give him a tool that's more satisfactory?" I argue. "And maybe some plastic ice cube trays?"

"He'd only ruin them, I'm sure. Wouldn't he, Len?"

"At least he'd have something to look at, something to do for a while," I try again.

"Not toys, no. Not toys, Poppa. He's just as well off this way."

"Nuzzin," says Mr. D.

"What was that, Poppa? Did you hear that, Len?"

"I think he said, Nothing," offers Len.

"No, he said something. I heard him say something. What did you say, Poppa?"

Mr. Danielson looks up fully for the first time, weary, dazed, uncomprehending: "Achesch itzerberrin."

"That's right, Poppa." Turning to me, Emily interpolates: "It's better just to repeat what he says."

"I think so too, Mr. Danielson," I answer. "After all, why not?" I am favored with a groan for my efforts.

"Itzerberrin," he shakes his head sagely.

"I just agree with this kind of doubletalk, I nod as though I understand him and he's right," she instructs me.

Suppose Mr. D. had just one flash of consciousness, of awareness? Suppose he's really with it all the time!?!

"Do you know who I am, Poppa?" Len leans over his father, peering close into his face. "Who am I, Poppa?"

If you don't know who you are, how should he, I want to scream.

"Do you think he knows us, Len? Poppa, who is this?"

"Bye-bye, Mr. Danielson," I wave to him. "I'll come see you next time, okay?" Mr. D.'s wrinkles rut his face till he's a sallow prune. He holds his head on one side, coyly, and curls his fingers together for the merest good-bye.

"Look at that, Len, he must think she's Anna. That's his niece," she elaborates, "who died, it's almost twenty-eight years ago. She always reminds him of Anna, I think. Don't you think so, Len?"

The voice fades away as I walk back to Dad's room.

# EIGHT

ON THANKSGIVING DAY, Mother takes a cab over to the nursing home. Her worried phone call interrupts me in the kitchen: "I think you'd better come over right away. Something's terribly wrong with Dad."

A little knot of nurses meets me at the top of the stairs.

"We can't figure it out. He tries to tell us, but—it's impossible. And yet, his voice sounds so peculiar, there seems to be an obstruction in his throat."

"Have you called the doctor?"

"Yes, he prescribed medication, but your father absolutely would not take it . . . Maybe he's smarter than we are . . . It *is* a holiday, you know. Dr. Mooney's on call, but only for emergencies."

They exchange guarded glances, then Mrs. Bellson stands taller and adds, "I know this is going to sound silly. But we've searched everywhere we can think of, we've gone through all the drawers in your father's room and looked all over the floor. We checked the linens and everything that's gone down to the laundry room, too. And we can't find them anywhere. If I didn't know better, I'd say he's swallowed his teeth!"

I try not to run, only to hurry. Mother is sitting on the edge of the bed, holding Dad's hand. He looks awful —greenish with red spots of fever spreading on his cheeks. Wasting no time on a greeting, pointing to his neck, Dad gurgles at us, "Teece, teece!"

I fly back to the nurses' station. "You're right! That's

what he's saying! He must have swallowed his teeth!"

"But it's impossible. A whole upper plate? It's so big—
the dentist made it specially that way so your dad'd be
able to manage it by himself. It can't be—he'd choke on
it immediately. And this has been going on since after
breakfast!"

Back we run to Dad's room; again he points at his
throat and at the nightstand drawer; we take out the
plastic case where his teeth usually reside, empty now.
"We understand, Dad. We'll get help." I pat his shoulder, and he nods in relief, eyes briefly fluttering toward
the ceiling.

We phone the doctor and he comes over immediately,
skeptical but professional. He examines Dad with shiny
instruments, shakes his head no, it's not possible, he
can't see a thing of importance down there in his throat.
He gives Dad a shot to quiet him, and goes back to his
holiday feast.

The afternoon wears on, and Dad waits, calmer, but
his breathing is labored, he's running a temperature,
and the gurgling noises are soupier. Detoured from our
holiday dinner, the whole family—kids too—assembles
at the nursing home to hold council. By three-thirty
everyone on the floor is as concerned as we. I pull the
short straw and am elected to call back the doctor, with
the hesitant but firm agreement of several nurses who
prefer to remain nameless.

"Dr. Mooney, I'm sorry to bother you again, but something *must* be done for Dad."

"Do you want X-rays taken?" he asks.

"If you think that's what should be done, yes. Of
course."

"Well, it's a holiday, but if you think it important enough, I'll have the technician come right over."

"Please do. And thanks."

"Call me when he gets there, and I'll tell him what to take."

We each pace a different territory of the halls, upstairs and down, waiting for the portable X-ray machine. When the man finally arrives, out of breath—he's alone on duty today—he phones the doctor, who obliges with instructions. The red-haired technician gently turns Dad about, recording his innards from several poses. Then, he informs us, he must go back to his office to develop the prints. He wheels his bulky apparatus through the reception room, where all the kids are gathered, glumly worried.

Dinnertime comes and goes; visitors, patients, nurses, and aides poke their heads in at the door, awed by this present installment. Dad is listless and sinking slowly, obviously. He refuses even a sip of water. It's after six when the doctor phones the desk at last, to report that nothing shows up on the X-rays.

My nephew, of junior-high age, is especially troubled. "Listen," he noticeably makes his decision to speak. "If Pop really *did* swallow his teeth, and they're probably made of some kind of plastic stuff, they won't show up on his stupid pictures anyway."

Back to the phonebooth for my final joust with Dr. Mooney: "Is it possible an upper plate wouldn't show up on the X-rays?"

"I suppose anything is possible," he counters smoothly. "But so far as I can see, there's nothing to go on here. What would you like me to do?"

"I don't know—that's supposed to be your business! Look. He doesn't want to live, and we don't want him to live either. But he just *can't* go this way, choking, slowly, all day, on his own teeth!! *Somebody* must do *something!*" I'm hot and cold and giggly and furious. "Wouldn't you consider this an emergency?"

"I don't think so. Do you think it is?" he asks calmly, accustomed to handling hysterical women like me. And, true, his answer is a smack in the face with a cold wet rag.

Our family panel is instantly unanimous: Dad cannot go like this; we must not let it happen in this ignoble manner. We phone a hospital (not in this district) for an ambulance, luckily reach a doctor who apparently deals with the exceptional in the manner of Marcus Welby, and who doesn't even repeat, "Swallowed his *what?*" when I pour out our story.

Dad is pale and quiet now, insists on being propped up as they pile him onto the stretcher. At the hospital they whisk him off efficiently, a pumplike gadget alerted for duty. By the time we've parked and spilled out into the proper waiting room, a young nurse whoops out of the room waving: "My God, look at the size of them! They came popping right out of his throat—I can't believe it! The ambulance ride must've dislodged 'em."

No tickertape, no rose petals. All the same, Dad is vindicated, he's a celebrity; everyone in the area who's mobile comes to rave over these teeth, and to smile and pat the cheek of the man in 217 who downed them.

He rests for a few days in the hospital, and then is transported back to Riverview, where he receives a hero's welcome. He settles back in his room with a

tearful, grateful, "I never could believe . . ." offering
for view his errant uppers.

At the end of the month I receive bills for the X-rays
and the extra visits made on Thanksgiving. I march into
Dr. Mooney's office and tell him as evenly as I can manage that we don't intend to pay in money too for the
agonies of that day. He holds out the pictures for my
appraisal, assuring both of us once more that there's no
indication of an obstruction.

"But even a fourteen-year-old knew that plastic
doesn't show up on X-rays!" I am losing the battle for a
businesslike tone of voice. "What would have happened
if we hadn't gotten him to the hospital where they believed him and suctioned his throat?"

"That might have been very sad," says the doctor,
fixing his face into an appropriate expression.

"You know what you can do with your goddamn pictures?" I shout. "You can . . . hang 'em on your wall
for your own private collection."

As I slam out the door, I'm bitterly pleased at Dr.
Mooney's shocked look. I'm sure he expected me to say
something quite different.

## NINE

NASTY WINTER WEATHER lasts only about three months in this part of the country, but the current season is interminable. We go on vacation. My husband needs about a week to unwind. I'm luckier: the minute I fasten my seat belt I'm on my way; by the time the stewardess asks what magazine we'd prefer, I'm unraveling. The tenth morning of our sunny reprieve we receive a cable: "Sad news. Dad passed away this morning." We reread it in disbelief, because it's signed by my husband's sister, not mine. It's *his* father who's died.

Back we come, thinking we must be on the funeral circuit of late. I take a martyr's pride at the number of deaths in our immediate families these past eighteen months: twelve. One by one, like playing card soldiers, uncles and aunts have gone—most of them with suddenness, all of them Dad's friends, all of them younger than he.

A snowy Sunday three weeks later we attend a funeral at 11 A.M., go out for a sandwich, then return to the parlor again at two. As the casket is wheeled in at the second service, a relative on my daughter's right whispers, "Poor Uncle Harry. He always hated going to funerals." On my left, my brother-in-law whispers back, "Well, he's sure coming to this one." Alicia and I grab one another's hands, leave the chapel in haste, handkerchieves stuffed at our mouths, many cousins surprised that we're this deeply affected. We rush to the ladies' room, choking on black laughter.

Very soon afterwards this same brother-in-law suffers a heart attack, and, by the time we reach the hospital, is no longer alive. The ironies pile up all around us, till we too are asking, Why? Has this family done something very wrong? During the mourning period, a thoughtful friend takes my sister's hand to comfort her: "You have, anyway, the consolation that your husband died like a gentleman." That's certainly a mind-boggler, but we forgo the opportunity of snagging the woman in further conversation. Apparently she thinks she means well.

Dad is so agitated when we tell him of his son-in-law's death, he thumps his chest and shakes his head violently from side to side with all his wretched strength, hoarsely crying out, "Me! Me! Not him! Me!" Mother bends tensely over him, the muscles above her jaws bulging. But she maintains a steady composure: "Try not to carry on so, dear. We just can't question these things."

A couple of weeks pass before my sister is able to face Dad. Fortunately no one requires us to determine whose anguish is the greater.

Another morning that same tormented winter, Mother stoops to pick up her knitting bag and falls, breaking her arm. We're all of the opinion she didn't slip, but rather toppled over from fatigue. Her biggest concern is not being able to visit Dad every day, so with logistical tidiness we deposit her in Riverview too to recuperate for a while. Her prime worry now is when she will be able to complete Afghan No. 51.

"How's everything going?" a friend phones to inquire.

"Well, we just got a great offer to sponsor ten half-hours. Lever Brothers heard we have lots of fresh material."

During her stay in the nursing home, Mother makes closer friends with some of the nurses, although they confide to us that it's sometimes a sticky business dealing with her: she's an exacting forelady whose consuming interest is only *one* of their patients. "They're too close, your mother and father," they warn us. "They're too dependent on one another; it's not wise."

These confidences spill over to include many of their own personal problems—disillusionment with marriage, an alcoholic husband, wayward kids, the usual—and a note of envy often insinuates into the conversations. For although Mother is the sole target of Dad's occasional outbursts of temper and frustration, she's able to treat such scenes with placid understanding until Dad is tearfully apologetic, bewildered at his own behavior, spent with self-hatred.

To many of the patients, Mother has become a sort of unofficial hostess—a Pearl Mesta of the aged—an unfailing daily visitor who presses a few after-dinner mints folded with a tissue into their waiting hands. They're surprised, some of them, at seeing her there full-time; they can't understand her role.

We don't find it easy either to distinguish among the others exactly who visits and who stays. For example, who belongs in Row A, and who in Row B:

The emaciated woman, blonde wig askew, with frightened, black-rimmed eyes and sparrow ways? (She's an aide. The kids name her Carrie the Ghoul.)

The woman who walks with a handsome, hale-and-hearty, athletic-shouldered husband, herself hobbling along on legs grotesquely bowed, a curious figure topped always by a flowered hat with pink or yellow veil, of 1940 vintage? (He's the patient; she's pushing him.)

The conscientiously grinning lady who often wears her clothes inside-out, always carries an empty shopping bag and a worn red change purse that she clicks open-shut, open-shut? (She's a pal of Martha from Room 39. She travels by train, subway, and bus to come here faithfully every other day. We had worried that she'd lost a serious amount of weight last July, slow to realize that she looked so different because she'd finally taken off her galoshes. Once a month her shopping bag is not so limp. It camouflages a bottle of gin and a jar of orange juice, which she and Martha guzzle and giggle over behind the barricaded door of Room 39.)

But momentary diversions are not enough: I must do more with my time and my life. While contemplating possibilities of my own little office . . . my own small business . . . the wheelchair concession at St. Petersburg Airport . . . a comic strip flash bulb appears over my head. The next balloon advises, "Don't think small. Start a big business. Open your own nursing home."

Seriously, why not? I could take over a motel near the ocean, shabby now, but with minor architectural changes, ideally suited. A quick count of the imminent needs of family and friends' families shows that I could be oversubscribed by the time the doorways were widened to stretcher size. This could be an exceptional residence, where the incapacitated could sociably re-locate with their more fortunate ambulatory spouses and friends. It would of course be a place for the old and the ill, but not a ghetto only for the hopelessly terminal. There could be housekeeping suites, where, for instance, Mother could bake while Dad looked on.

It's such a super idea, I begin writing copy:

> Are you bedridden, sisters? Can't get yourselves up, brothers? Well, why not just groove with the pain! Don't take old age lying down—swing into senility at Funnyfarm in Happy Acres. This may not be where it's at, but it sure is where it gets to.

The *New York Times* may insist on a less facetious tone, but I can adapt.

When I take my proposition to our accountant, he reels off a long list of problems insurmountable to one as naïve as I, highlighted by the fact that the whole thing is not financially viable. I sigh over the decision to keep the accountant and scrap the plan.

I get a job instead.

## TEN

MOTHER IS TORN, leaving Dad at Riverview, but joyous
to return home, arm mending nicely. An obscure fairy
instructs one Mrs. Reinert to answer our ad in the paper
for part-time housekeeper/companion, and we snatch
her up on the spot. Of a soon-to-be-extinct breed is our
Mrs. Reinert. With all her life juices, she believes there's
not an inanimate object in the world that should escape
scouring, waxing, polishing, washing, starching, ironing,
boiling, or at least soaking in Clorox. The animate may
elude her but are made to feel ostracized. Though with
proper formality they are never to progress to a first-
name basis, Mrs. Reinert and Mother are instantly, continually delighted with one another. We make an
arrangement with Circle Cabs for Mother's daily transportation to the nursing home, and I get swallowed up
by the International Association of Urban Institutes,
Mr. Schlossberg's Office. (The steno isn't bad, but what
a mouthful identifying him on the telephone!) And the
seasons straggle on.

A new patient is brought in to occupy the room next
to Dad's. We are introduced, with deserved reverence,
to a stately, clear-skinned Mother Superior, nearly blind
and, 'tis said, with a very short time left on mortal ter-
rain. This being the first time Mother Agatha has spent
any appreciable time away from her convent in over
fifty years, scores of people come to see her—family and
friends who can at last visit without restriction. Im-

mersed in socializing, she adores every contact during these waning months. Soon my mother is bringing two portions of soup and applesauce and sponge cake, and Mother Agatha blossoms under the change of regimen and diet.

A sunny morning shortly after her arrival, in the bathroom connecting her room with Dad's, the folds of her habit are caught behind the john. The Mother Superior is forced to lean over most ungracefully to push open the door and call to Dad to please ring for the nurse. That neither of them is particularly embarrassed over the incident is divine; Dad, Mother, and the nun are thus thereafter bound in friendship.

For Dad, life begins to go downhill. Every few weeks he suffers a spell, a spasm, an attack, an infection, a virus, a little stroke perhaps. Actually he's not strong enough for a thorough examination, our new doctor informs us, all the while pumping him full of B-12 and assorted body-builders. After each setback Dad is a tiny bit weaker, his speech further impaired; drop by drop he ebbs, till we can't imagine how much more can be left of his strength to endure. Never, ever does it occur to us that it will be his wanton fate to continue this way for several years.

"He must have a very strong heart," says a commiserating sage.

"Not really. He's had a slight heart condition for about twenty-five years," I correct the record.

"Did he ever have high blood pressure?"

"Well, no. It was always low."

"He never drank at all, did he? But he always used a lot of salt on his food . . ."

"Matter of fact, Dad always had a drink or two before dinner, so long as we can remember. And what does salt have to do with anything?"

"I thought perhaps . . . Well, the bed rest all these years has undoubtedly strengthened him. That's the way the cookie crumbles, I guess."

"Why?"

"What'd you say? I didn't hear you."

"Oh, sorry. Yeah, that is the way it sometimes crumbles."

❀    ❀    ❀

The phone calls have come during a slow Sunday brunch, while we're at a friend's home for the evening, just as I'm opening the door with an armful of groceries. This time I am at work when Mrs. Bellson reaches me: "I think you'd better come over, and maybe call your sister too. Dad isn't doing well at all."

1. Alert my husband
2. Phone my sister
3. Drop everything else
4. Run

The sympathetic Mr. Schlossberg is getting to know the pattern well; he wishes me luck as I leave the office.

In the car I wonder what I would do if it were snowing and I'd just washed my hair. I don't own a hat, and have never gone out the door in rollers-and-clips. Would I take time to dry it well, or encase my head in Saranwrap and fly? I'm tense about driving and visualizing the "arrangements" that I morbidly hope will have to be made. With disconcerting practicality, I regret that I have only one simple black dress, winter-weight and too warm for now. I can never decide whether it's more maudlin to buy an extra funereal type outfit to hold in abeyance, or to anticipate shopping for one in haste. What do other people do if, like me, they don't usually wear black? Can one start family gossip going by wearing navy blue? I recall a hairdresser who, while trimming my hair, bent close to my ear to tell me that the woman who'd just come in for a shampoo and set had lost her husband the night before.

When I arrive at Riverview Mrs. Bellson stops me at the desk: "It's amazing. We think it must've been another stroke, and we surely thought you wouldn't get here in time. But he's rallied now, and we're going to give him some broth for dinner. Sorry to bring you over again for a false alarm."

"No demerits this time," I assure her as I go down the hall.

Pale as his pillow, Dad looks up, questioning why I should be there in the middle of a working day.

"They told me you weren't doing so well, Dad," I hope to be casual. "How's it now?"

"No good," he answers weakly, staring at me intently. Pointing to my forehead, he adds, "Nu."

Mother and I exchange puzzled looks, then, what a relief to laugh out loud. I've worn new eyeglasses for three days now, and he's the first person to notice.

Mother tells me quietly, "I'm sorry we dragged you away from your office, but things looked so bad. I was afraid he was almost . . . but those nurses are wonderful, really. They ran in here with all their equipment and got to work so quickly. They are just marvelous. They used it for only a very short while, and then he pulled out of it so well they didn't need it any more." Dad concentrates on her hand as she pats the oxygen tank. From depths of weariness and disdain, he asks of it, "Why? Why? Why!!!" Calmer, then, he completes his question: "Why am I alive?"

The Mother Superior cautiously taps on the door, and we welcome the interruption. "I've been praying for you, Matthew."

"That's very kind of you, Mother Agatha."

So *she's* the one!

A weird process is going on here, and I am not privy to its council. An R&D study might be wise . . . A little late for anybody Up There to get to know about me, but possibly I could arrange for equal time. After all, I haven't tried it, so I shouldn't knock it.

## ELEVEN

"Honey! How *are* you?" An admonishing arm encircles Michael's waist. "You've lost a little weight, haven't you?"

My nephew Michael and I are caught at the nursing home when some old family friends arrive to see Dad. They cluster around the bed, presenting themselves in turn, and Dad kisses their hands in greeting. They are well-intentioned, kind; only their own sudden collapse— and how they would love describing such an event!— would keep them from visiting the first Sunday of every month. After a few amenities, they rapidly zero in on the subject of Michael's hair. (We also rely on his long curls, his unironed work shirt, and torn, patched, embroidered jeans: the young generation's uniform provides unending wonderment for Dad.)

Looking around eagerly to snare any potential listener—finding one or finding none—they each subside into separate conversations, delivered simultaneously.

Dad tries to concentrate on:

I can't complain, really. But I had to go to the ear doctor three times last week for this infection. You know, the boil I had behind my ear, well, you would never in your life believe such a size. And it was so painful when the doctor had to lance it. Of course I went to a specialist—he's the top man at City Hospital. They can't give you any anesthetic for that kind of thing, you know. It's a good thing I didn't faint in his office; it's always so crowded,

there's no room to fall down. Never in my life have
I gone through such an ordeal! But how can I complain?

which is spoken at the same time as:

The other day I went to see my Aunt Sally. She's
going to be seventy-six next month, bless her. My
nephew Peter—I don't think you know him, but
you don't know Sally either, do you? Anyway,
Peter and Jeannie called for me, and Evelyn Barnes
and her two children were in the car. Evelyn's
a cousin of Ruth and Paul's—they used to be
neighbors of ours. Anyway, what a scrap they
all had in the car, all the way out there! Unbeliev-
able. Anyway, Aunt Sally had just gotten back
from Florida, where she went to rest up after visiting in L.A. with Rob and Barbara. From there of
course she had to go to San Francisco to see Ellie
and Artie. I don't think you ever met any of her
children, did you? Anyway, you have to hand it to
Aunt Sally. She can't stand to sit still in one place
for long. She does hate to stay put.

Michael and I can't look at Dad, whose attention, anyway, is sought by the third speaker:

It got to the point where I absolutely had to tell
her off, the woman who is *supposed* to be my superior. Naturally she got where she is by being
friendly with . . . the point being . . . Well, the
standards of achievement in every field today are
certainly something else again. Nobody cares about
a proper day's work or anything well done. It's just
impossible the way they take their . . . You know,
their coffee breaks are more important than the job
at hand. Craftsmanship is a thing of the past, and
we are all suffering . . . the point being . . .

while, in counterpoint,

> Trying to find a parking space around here is really impossible. Do you know how long it took me to ride around and around the block? Have you any idea? Just try to guess—take a guess. It's such a ridiculous situation, I tell you, they're going to have to do something about it . . .

is trying to be heard.

Sudden laughter from the fastest talker: "When you finish with that, *I* have a story for you." Then, turning to Michael without breaking stride, "Honey, aren't you feeling well?"

"Me? I'm fine. Why?"

"You're so quiet . . ."

Dad flutters his hand in tolerant defeat. He is most assuredly a captive audience, but how much he can decipher from the din is hard to calculate. For these people are Tolstoy rejects—part of that lonely lunatic fringe who talk at one another, often of anecdotes from a past never dead to them, of arguments with a disagreeable salesclerk or nasty streetcar conductor. (How long ago could *that* one have taken place, when it's over thirty years since the trolley tracks were torn up?) The incidents were inconsequential when they originally took place; still the dialogue can be repeated today—and repeated and repeated—verbatim.

Michael and I snatch at the momentary sanctuary of a water cooler around the bend of the hall.

"Jesus! ! ! I forgot all about those crazies!" Michael, home from a year at college, clutches his head as if to secure it, hair included. "How does Pop stand it?!"

## TWELVE

PEOPLE HAD ALWAYS been surprised to learn that Dad was a tavern owner who tended his own bar: he wasn't the type. Shy, with a quiet fund of knowledge astonishing for his four years of schooling, he never drank with the customers, and preferred "darn" to "damn."

On Sundays and holidays, when he worked a double shift—from noon till 2 A.M.—Mother would carefully pack a "picnic" lunch and dinner of sandwiches, hot soup, coffee, cookies, and extra napkins, which my sister and I took turns bringing to him. We had to go around to the side door because females weren't allowed in taverns in those days. The customers, many of them steadies since before we were born, were lined up at the long bar polished to a mirror. Everything else was dark, smoky wood and the smell of beer.

"Here's your daughter, Matt. And let's see what the good woman has sent you today."

"Come on, dearie, have a pretzel."

"Holy Christ, Matt, are you gonna eat all that?"

Dad would wipe his hands carefully and come to take the brown paper bag, with a slight smile and a shrug of, Don't mind them, they're all right. His long white apron would be spotless. I don't ever remember seeing his hands dirty either; in the winter his knuckles were so chapped from washing, they would bleed.

My sister and I used to hate Sundays and holidays; everybody else's family was off relaxing. At home,

Mother would bake or sew or read or something; she'd never go to the movies with us, she'd wait till Dad could go too. Our family took only one vacation together, when I was four or five. We drove up to Niagara Falls and then out to Ohio someplace to visit with relatives on a farm.

"Dad and I don't need vacations the way other people seem to," Mother always said. "On his day off, we are very happy just to go to a movie."

"But all the other kids go on vacations," we would whine.

"Let them do what they do; you be different." (Another way of saying, "We can't afford it.")

My parents were fond of recalling a few special treats, when they'd indulged in two double features with a light dinner in-between.

❊　❊　❊

Now holidays, birthdays, and anniversaries are still difficult; but we're all determined to deal with them via cookies, champagne in paper cups, and a lightness of spirit. As for gifts—how many kinds of hard candies and mints are there? How many patterns of pajamas? When the heel on his old slipper wears through (from shuffling his "good" foot about while he sits in his chair), we buy new ones for Dad, in a dilemma about how to offer— how to giftwrap—half a pair. Solution: Make the replacement, unobtrusively, in his closet, saying nothing of the switch. Down to the incinerator with the super-fluous right-footed scuff.

For his eighty-second birthday we bring a "Pin It On, Pop" bulletin board for snapshots; at his eighty-third, a small magnifying glass in a black leather case. We gloat over the inspirations of a Gro-Light for the wrought-iron plant stand, and a tank with five goldfish. Two lively Fathers' Days are spent setting these up. On their fifty-fourth anniversary—the fourth celebrated in this room—we present a lamp with two revolving shades; as they turn, geometric figures swirl hypnotically.

We tape to the walls photos of a grandson, proud in graduation gown and cowl; glamorous poses of Alicia with thick honey hair almost as long as her mini-skirt. "I can go bra-less; it's the fashion, you know, Pop," she explains. "And nobody can tell because my hair covers that much of me." Too bad Dad's blood pressure is so low: how he must ache to reward her with a proud blush!

We "Contact" the top window pane, giving a stained glass authenticity to Mother Agatha's daily blessings. Friends send tokens of their travels: a gay wall hanging from Mexico, Israeli dancers on a round brass plaque, a colorful glass owl to hold the windowshade in place.

When the plastic electric clock falls off the nightstand in a final spin, we substitute a digital clock, hoping that the turning numbers might add a patch of intrigue to Dad's long dozing-on-and-off nights. Next day, adamant, he demands of it: "Home! Out! Go!"

"Why don't you like it, Dad?" we ask, but his explanation is a furious jumble of consonants we're never able to figure out.

I put the clock at my side of our bed, and coincidentally (or as a result?) have a sleepless night of my own soon afterward. I wake with a start at one fifty-eight, to the tune of "Two minutes to two, two minutes more to say 'I love you.'" At one-fifty-nine I realize that the song goes "One minute to one." Undaunted, George Raft continues to Peabody over a moon-lit parquet floor with a graceful, unknown blonde. Two fifteen becomes two and a quarter: the old auctioneer can hardly wait till two and a half rolls around so he can chant over the radio, "A-ling-a-ling-a-ling-a-Sold American." Was 314 my homeroom in senior high school? Or was it 319? . . . By this time I think I understand why Dad objected so to these tireless digits, dispassionately, ever so slowly, flopping one's life into oblivion.

We offer instead a wall clock, hanging it near the door where he can easily see it. Now there are so many electrical gadgets on that side of the room, we have to get a third extension cord, and wander about searching for another outlet. When Dad realizes what we're looking for, he makes us understand somehow that there's one on the baseboard behind his bed.

"How in the world did you know it was there, Dad?" From his chair, and certainly from bed, he can't possibly see that part of the room.

"Dunno," he answers.

He points and motions patiently from one plug to the other, till we see that we can apportion an equal number into each socket. Meanwhile about his head echoes the kids' ever-confident phrase from way back: "Pop'll fixit."

❖   ❖   ❖

Our older daughter Susan is to be married, and the flurry of happy details overrides all else. She presents her young man to Dad, who gravely nods approval, seeing well beneath the shaggy black beard and sandals. On another visit she ducks into the ladies' room and out of sneakers and jeans, to give a private prevue of how she will look as a bride. Dad examines especially the white silk shoes, the creamy bow that holds her veil. Then, tearfully, he holds her hand, exacting over each syllable: "I am very happy."

The wedding is bittersweet for Mother, unaccompanied, to attend. "I don't know how I do it, how I can laugh and talk to people," she shakes her head in sad wonder, "knowing that Dad is lying there like that. I must be made of iron."

We bring back flowers and a piece of Mother's triumphant homemade chocolate wedding cake. And, later on, the pictures, which claim a prominent place on the crowded walls of his domain.

# THIRTEEN

RIVERVIEW'S MIDNIGHT STAFF spreads the story, and we learn of an entry logged in the night records of March 7, 1971. Mother Agatha shyly corroborates; we imagine the details.

A soft, brushing noise, scrape of a hinge, and Dad looks up at the scalloped kitchen clock, out of place here but with clear luminous hands. Is it five of three or quarter past eleven? What is disturbing the monotony of another dreamless night? He reaches for the bedrail and pulls himself over slightly, hazy about the wobbly shadow shuffling out of the connecting bathroom. He remembers that his john-mate is the Mother Superior, but she never gets up at night alone, and with propriety has never entered his room through that door.

The shape inches its way nearer Dad's bed, silhouetted against a sudden light from Mother Agatha's room. He makes out a curly white head, sunglasses, a big grin. Barefoot, bony-kneed, the figure holds aloft what seems at first a torch; then, more clearly, his bell jar with catheter still attached and coiling about his waist and hips, disappearing under the white muslin hospital gown. Mother Agatha apparently had an unexpected caller who wandered through her room and into his.

Dad's habitual gallantry surfaces. He motions angrily at the man, and as loudly as he can manage, shouts, "Go! Go home!" He falls back on the pillow, easing his shoulder around till he's able to reach the other rail.

Doubling back his hand, he rings for the nurse. His room fills with one nurse, two, an aide, an orderly—enjoyable commotion. All unbelieving laughter, they steer the man back to his own bed, an even more unlikely Diogenes from the rear with his bare, flabby buttocks.

"Tell 'em to be careful!" he requests of Dad. "Tell 'em to watch what they're doin' with them balls! Hear, now: my balls are very precious to me!"

As the procession leaves his room, Dad chuckles as best he can. Then wonders perhaps: Where am I?

## FOURTEEN

MOTHER AGATHA has her priorities; I am thankful for music. Dad and Mother have always enjoyed listening, with truly catholic taste. They also instilled in us the highest regard for our Mason & Hamlin, the instrument we were never allowed to approach with unclean hands. Nobody ever heard Dad sing, but he whistled often and well; never did he try to dance a step, possibly because his feet were so flat and he was self-conscious about them. Mother told us that when they were first married, they'd gone to the Broadway Central where an irresistible dance band played through the dinner hour. Dad had rather formally presented himself to a group of soldiers at a nearby table, asking whether one of them wouldn't like to dance with his wife, who was longing to join the others on the floor. Mother'd had several lovely waltzes this way, with Dad nodding admiringly from the sidelines.

He loved to listen to us practice the piano. Though he dozed behind his newspaper, we knew he could spot every mistake. When the hour was up, he'd rouse from the armchair and say, "That was beautiful," graciously including the hateful, uneven scales.

Since he's been confined, we've tried many times to leave a radio on his nightstand, but he will never allow it—nor will he listen to a musical TV program. On Mothers' Day, scrounging for a novelty, we bring the tape recorder and set it on his tray table. For this in-

troductory session we've taped "The Nutcracker Suite,"
and are relieved when, with no objection, Dad relaxes
into the music as it becomes familiar.

"Hoozizh?" he asks, pointing from one reel to the
other.

"Tchaikovsky wrote this." I have no notion if that's
the question he has in mind.

"You know, Pop," adds one of the kids, "Tchaikovsky
was a Russian, and he composed this about a hundred
years ago. He wrote such beautiful music, but his life
was very sad."

"Jewish?" asks Dad, plainly this time.

"No, but he had other troubles. He had a nervous
breakdown and he was a homosexual."

Mother raises a disapproving head: "I didn't think
they knew about such things!" Then she sighs, "Or
maybe they just never talked about it so much in those
days."

Our musicale is such a success, I depend on the tape
recorder when I can't otherwise propel myself into
cheerfulness at the top of those steamy stairs. Every
few weeks I bring: Beethoven, for perspective; Brahms,
for dwarfing these surroundings and this mission; Benny
Goodman, for a short, ludicrous jam session; Chopin,
with a reminder of Arthur Rubinstein bouncing up and
down on the piano bench. Playing a tape of early Ella
and Satchmo, I report that Louis Armstrong is seriously
ill now. Dad listens attentively to this one, then cries
long and very hard.

Embedded in nostalgia are the selections that make
one weep. Mother welled up recently hearing "My
Hero" on the radio, recalling her eldest brother, dead

some thirty years. He'd sung it in their Social Circle
Club's *Chocolate Soldier*, performed sixty years ago to
raise money for the town's underpriviledged—at that
date poor—people . . . My sister had to excuse herself
with a sob from a dinner table because "Smoke Gets in
Your Eyes" brought a stingingly fresh realization of her
husband's death . . . I always cry at weddings when
"Here Comes the Bride" is played, even if she's chubby
or perspiring. The sole exception: when it was ac-
companied by the release of plastic doves, which zoomed
on invisible cords crisscrossing the ceiling of Bridal
Chapel No. Five, Herrold's Ceremonial Halls, Avenue
H, Brooklyn, 10526 . . .

One grey Sunday our Riverview concert includes
the score from a musical Dad had especially enjoyed.
During "Some Enchanted Evening" two little women
interrupt their endless strolling around the halls to
hover at the doorway, nudging each other as though
they must settle an urgent dispute. The skinny blonde
witchlike one finally detaches herself and enters with
determination. Squinting moistly into Dad's face, she
says, "You're remarkable. You're wonderful. Why didn't
you tell us you could sing?"

Rather than attempt a reply, Dad offers the kind lady
a choice of M&Ms or miniature sour balls.

*     *     *

A few days later, while watching a Halo commercial
with mother, Dad stiffens abruptly, his head falling to
his chest. Mother runs for the nurse, and a battery of
professionals hurry in with emergency trappings. When
I arrive, Mrs. Bellson tells me, "He seems to be popping

out of it again, but I really don't know . . ." Then, apologetically, "I know your father doesn't want to live—we can *all* understand when he tells us *that*. But we just have to do what we have to do. Maybe this time, if your mother hadn't been there . . . Anyway, we brought in the oxygen tank, and he fought it so, we finally wheeled it out again. When I took it away he kissed my hand over and over." She busies herself at the desk. "You know, he's the only man who ever kissed my hand . . ."

In his room, Mother is leaning back in the chair, still and aged, with nothing much to say. For many years now it has been suggested that her own long history of illness and surgery may have been rooted in "keeping it all inside." But, she once said, "What do you do to get it all out? How should I go about doing that?"

I kiss Dad's forehead. "How's it going, Dad?"

He barely opens an eye. "Please," he whimpers, at last displacing his favored, "Why?"

After dinner I go back to the nursing home, drawn toward the drama of this struggle with life. I sit by the bed, and, taking his hand, realize that with my thumb and second finger I can circle his wrist with an alarming amount of space to spare. No nursing expertise is needed to recognize that his is a worrisome pulse: it machine-guns, flutters to a stop, hammers away fiercely, halts not quite completely. With breathing to match. Slipping into consciousness for a few moments, he looks slowly, with wistful finality, all about the darkened room, as if to engrave on his memory every picture and plant, every companionable object.

Why are sickrooms always shadowed? To entice sleep to tempt death? Because the dying might be additionally discomfited to see clearly that they are indeed dying? (Perhaps they'd rather view as distinctly as possible a dear, final, still available sight.) Or because the sensibilities of the spectators are eased by a softened twilight? In the sharp fluorescence of an operating room, should a clumsy or incautious surgeon nick too deeply, do the lights lower automatically as the victim's breathing ceases?

Yes. Optimally, one should die in dimness, but not in the dark.

I sit there a long time, shivering, not daring to look away from my father's face, attempting to induce his reprieve: "Now. Stop. Now. Die. Sleep. Now." I'm silently hysterical when I hear myself think, "Please!"

At quarter past nine he responds to an inner alarm bell, shifts slightly, and gradually remembers who I am. He lazily sorts over the items coursing through his mind, selects one that he feels he can verbalize: "Mudder home?"

I assure him that Mother's okay and that he will be too. With an effort he brings my hand to his lips for a good-night kiss, then lapses into semi-sleep without noticing how the nightstand is placed, how many Kleenex are folded over the sheet, whether the bell is tied on the rail. Perhaps release is near: he doesn't look toward the door as I leave.

On my way home I ponder over what music to bring, should Dad pull through once more and we're visiting on future Sundays. If I were to prepare a record, a carefully varied medley, I could maybe become rich and famous. It could certainly be a hit in the nursing home market. I would entitle this album "Music To Die By."

✿    ✿    ✿

Next morning before going to work I check in on Riverview. Forced to avow he's vaguely recovering, Dad
motions to the tank, where one of the goldfish floats life-
lessly. He flutters a distracted fist at his chest, straining
to sound out, "Me! Me!" While the four other fish swim
about unconcernedly, insensitive to their loss and to
ours.

## FIFTEEN

THE PAST COUPLE of weeks have not been good, so my husband and I flee to a deserted motel for the weekend. We never fight, my husband and I. Rather, we get quiet, withdrawn, distant from one another, sometimes for days. Then, at a hopeful mutual signal, we talk.

This time, as we walk on the sand, I persist in asking what's bugging him, unprepared for the array he tosses out like polite daggers. He enumerates calamitous business woes, but brushes them away in company with his lousy backhand in tennis. The larger problem emerges. Without recrimination, without blame—he feels as much at fault for allowing it—we have become so dominated by the situation with my parents that we do little that deeply pleases us.

"What makes you so actively interested in your parents?" he asks me one of those simple, impossible questions.

"I guess I have no choice—I'm of the same stuff they are."

"And why do you keep visiting?" That one, too, I'd prefer to be rhetorical.

"Must be responsibility that keeps me at it. Everybody has to have something to hang on to. I really do think life is meaningless, but maybe I can make it seem less meaningless . . ."

Yuk, yuk, yuk. I remember the one about the lady in the asylum who runs around with no clothes on, only a hat and gloves. She wears no clothes because nobody ever comes to see her. She wears the hat and gloves because somebody *might* come.

"I'd never be this involved if it were my own family," he says after a while, putting his arm around my shoulders to steer me down to harder packed sand. "But I understand that you must be, and in a way I'm glad."

For a few steps I wear a glorious halo of Commitment, but it rightfully slides down over my nose in the ocean wind.

"As long as it hurts, it's better to hurt a little more," a masochistic streak informs me privately. So I force open the issue of having to pay for all this in money, too. (Fortunately, oh how fortunately, my husband earns enough to support these staggering bills; Dad's savings had run out shortly after the first year. I've asked a lot of people, who supply knowing, conspiratorial glances, but no straightforward information about how the not-so-affluent manage.)

"Okay, if you want to talk about the money part of it, we can, but it's not a very productive topic. Anyhow, I really don't know how much each item costs. One day, I suppose, I'll get belted with it." He digs a silly face out of the sand with his toe. "Like transporting your mother back and forth, and flour and sugar for all that therapeutic baking. And the drug bill, for instance."

"You know what the doctor told me the other day when I asked what all those prescriptions were? He told me one of them is to help prevent Dad from getting pneumonia, but he already has emphysema and might get it anyhow. He said it would be better if Dad just went to sleep and didn't wake up. So I asked why we couldn't help do just that. He got furious with me—said he'd *deport* me for acting on such a suggestion. Maybe I should take him up on the offer . . . I'm pretty stupid. I forgot he's a part owner of the nursing home and must get about two dollars a minute every time he visits."

My husband's cartoon gets five toes of curly bangs. "I don't know . . . As long as we can afford it without getting too much in a hole, and neither of us cares that you're not up to your eyebrows in ermine, I guess we just do it. Somehow I can't quite see us putting them on Welfare."

When I write the monthly checks, I mentally lop off the last one or two digits, figuring only in tens. I am a slavey keeping someone else's books, never looking back over the stubs. I place before me a double shot of whisky, in case I contemplate disposing otherwise of these funds, and start to guess how many gifted students could attend, and riot against, the college of their choice . . . how many families could live decently per annum . . . how I would look in a few of Liz Taylor's jewels . . what size Greek island could be bought, with ten percent off for cash . .

Over a barrel the nursing home's got us. Over a barrel endlessly rolling. Does anyone listen to the complaints of a Welfare patient who can't talk? Emotional blackmail—that's what it is: We have to keep up with the payments so we can feel lucky if we get our money's worth of caring care.

I stop to shake a shell off my foot. "I sort of think of us as part of the Economy of Obsolescence. We're big consumers. It's ironic, since we both hate to go shopping."

"And I imagine that when we're finally through with this whole business, I'll probably be incapacitated, financially and physically. We'll both be worn out, emotionally and sexually. The final irony will probably be that I won't be able to do too much more with my own life."

## AND DAD KNOWS IT ALL

streams across the sky like an advertising banner waving from a low-flying plane.

We let a mile of sand exhaust us.

I picture Dad when I'd seen him the other day. Mother had been out of the room briefly, dispensing peppermints, and he'd clutched at my hand, pleading directly with me, clearly for once, "Please, my dear, get rid of me." I recall an acquaintance who'd swallowed a hundred aspirin and not quite accomplished what she'd set out to do. One hundred twenty-five speedier Bufferin should do the deed—for me, that is. But what about Dad? Again, this ugly riddle. I loathe this game. I always lose. Somebody else always picks up all the marbles.

"Meanwhile, my darling," my husband interrupts my reverie, "enough of this bloody sand, let's get the hell back to our room. We didn't come here *only* to depress ourselves . . . You get out the booze and I'll go for the ice, and who knows? With a little bit of luck we may even be able to stagger along your ocean again later, and see if the waves are still rolling in like we taught them to."

Let the liberated ladies raise their consciousnesses, let them levitate en masse: I would go down on my knees nightly for this man. More realistically, I might let him beat me at Scrabble.

* * *

We hate to leave the lovely anonymity of our two-day retreat, but as we near the city I'm perversely impatient with the slow miles, thinking about the Jerusalem cherry tree that Mother has been tending since she brought it from the nursing home more than three years ago. Scraggly and frail at first, it had grown lush and full under her care, flourishing over sizable cubic footage in a room without much natural light, breathing city fumes miles from its customary habitat. Several times pale green berries had formed, only to drop off before turning their cheerful red, amid a shower of leaves. Mother had fed it vitamins and coaxed it along, and each time it renewed itself with surprising vigor.

One such misery had befallen the little tree shortly before Dad's last siege. Inexplicably, they had both recovered.

The other night I had remained in Dad's room when two nurses came to straighten the bed. (Usually we wait outside, in deference to his continuing modesty.) As they pulled him up onto the pillow, the blanket pushed aside, revealing for an instant a part of the skeletal torso—yellowed, like withered leaves—for which he no longer had any respect.

This knack that Mother has with plants: perhaps that's what's keeping him alive too. A while ago, transplanting the cherry bush for the third time, she hadn't pushed it far enough into the soil to cover the roots completely. (Psychology at work—or couldn't she see them well enough?) Still, it had grown to preside over the whole of the corner table, allowing no one to sit on the slice of couch before it.

Just before we'd left the city Friday night, Mother had been upset to see that lots of leaves had once again faded and begun to fall off. She'd added more plant food, watered and turned it, and worried over its fate.

I can't wait till we open the door at home—to see how that Matthew Tree is faring, and to find out whether the head nurse has called.

## SIXTEEN

THESE UPS AND DOWNS are wearing for us; how they can be for Dad is unimaginable. We sometimes think it would be easier if he were not still mentally alert; tempered with this is the recollection that he had always considered disease of the mind the worst of all afflictions, more fearful than blindness. It's agonizing that there's no language available to him to hint at what's been occupying his mind these long, desolate years—that he can't tell us whether a docile unawareness might after all be preferable to his unintelligible limbo. Why should this be his particular destiny? Could it be that he's breaking some Kafkaesque rule by remaining a thinking, responsive person? That he may achieve no real peace until he's been thoroughly crushed into predetermined components of senility and bitterness?

Is he aware that he averages seven comprehensible words per afternoon, and therefore experiments with his limited supply of sounds—vowels on Mondays, Wednesdays, Fridays; consonants, the balance of the week—trusting they'll emerge as rehearsed? Or is he incapable of such organization, since "planning" maddeningly demands that he be there the next day, and the next? No matter. However he may try to enlarge his repertoire, all distinguishable inquiries distill into: "Wha' day?" "How's chillun?" "Wukking?" and "How're you?"

With kindness and clarity he does say, every day be-

tween four thirty and five, "Get ready; go home." Does
he issue that directive because he senses that each of us
is wearier of Riverview even than he? Or because he's
eager to indulge in the secret store of remembrances
that he's lined up for the night? (When I ascribe for my
father any glimmer of salvation, or interest, within his
circumstance, I feel especially guilty for hours.)

In the beginning, he used to try to talk with us. He
would seemingly ask a question, and we'd lean closer
and say, "What was that, Dad? I didn't quite get that,"
or "I didn't hear you." He'd make elaborate attempts to
be distinct, but the words would spill out like vocal
Silly Putty. These would be dreaded scenes; as a result
he's been quieter the past few years.

When Dad does initiate a conversation, we resort to a
combination of Charades and Twenty Questions to decipher what he's saying. Though from the resigned
flagging of his hand—that "Oh, never mind, what's the
use?" gesture—we know that most often we're far from
his subject. I might vamp a few um-humhs when he
pauses; but if he's asking for information rather than a
yes/no reply—or if he's not asking a question at all!—
he looks at me levelly and I am caught, floundering to
mask our shared dismay. If my answer should accidently
fall into the right arena, Mother asks, "What did he
say? You seem to understand him better." And I must
move where I hope Dad can't see me and semaphore to
Mother. I can never satisfactorily explain to her that I
am equally confused—just more practiced in the non-
committal garblings of parlor talk.

Impossible to tally the man-hours spent trying to
decode: Have you lost your earring, or neglected to put
on the second one? . . . Check the middle drawer for

molasses mints that the night orderly prefers . . . You've lost a button off your coat sleeve . . . A clean towel was issued today, but no washcloth . . . You're forgetting to feed the fish . . . The umbrella you left yesterday has been put in a corner of the closet for safekeeping.

Most torturous are the countless communiqués we never understand at all.

So we try to choose a theme first, babbling on to keep the chatter flowing. For example, I report that the local supermarket was robbed over the weekend. Dad is unaccountably interested in the details, so I fabricate till my imagination balks. Still, he continually refuses to look at a paper or watch a news program. Possibly he doesn't know who our current president is. (Then again, maybe he's spared unhappiness on that score at least.) We do force him to see on TV that men are playfully bounding over the surface of the moon—the same moon he hasn't seen in over five years. But we're uncertain he grasps what a giant step has been taken. How he would have been riveted to the set in easier times!

✿   ✿   ✿

Visitors have dwindled to a faithful few. "Speedy recovery" mail has stopped altogether. Now there's only an occasional "Thinking of You" message or a postcard from vacationing friends. Mother of course continues to go every day. Early in the winter she confesses to several "weak spells" she's had at the nursing home, her cantankerous heart furious at the tasks she's been forcing on it. Dad, she says, makes immediate diagnosis, and motions her to a chair, pointing to her handbag and his mouth, indicating she must count on her nitros to discharge their duties "every thirty seconds as needed."

(Mother does wonder if she might eventually blow up from an accumulation.)

"You should phone Mrs. Bellson before you leave home, and she'll have the porter open the emergency gate for your cab. Then you won't have to climb that long flight of stairs." My sister and I are insistent.

"I don't like to bother them, they're very busy at two o'clock," counters Mother.

"They won't mind, they've said you should do that."

"No, I'd rather not . . . Anyhow, what's the difference? If it comes, it comes. If I go, I go." Reasonable, matter-of-fact, she reaches into her knitting bag for a measuring tape.

I see my mother reincarnate: She's a parachute tester. She's a lady matador who prefers a freshly crocheted afghan to a cape. In reverse drag, she competes in an all-male marathon roller derby. She's the first tour guide on Venus, awaiting arrival of an overdue Bar Mitzvah group.

She agrees to visit Dad three hours a day instead of four.

She arrives at Riverview on St. Patrick's Day to find him sitting in his chair, crying, unusually despondent. His relief at seeing her is enormous. Mother is horrified at his dilemma: there's a roach on his leg, crawling at leisure in and out the folds of his pajamas. He can't reach over to swat at it, he can't move his "good" leg far enough to brush it away, he can't reach the bell from his chair. He has to just sit there, watch it, and wait for help.

In an effort to divert him, Mother reminds him of favorite jokes they used to laugh at; she seizes on anything she can think of to rechannel his thoughts. She gets out the albums we've made in a "This Is Your Life" mode. "Good heavens! Just see how heavy I was on our twenty-fifth anniversary! I think I look younger today. . . I'm sorry I never gave you a son," she says. "Have you missed not having a boy?"

Dad just looks at her sweetly, pats her hand.

Later that evening, Mother says, "It's heartbreaking. He's such a lovable person. What could he have done to deserve such punishment?"

What, indeed? I find comfort in listing greater tragedies that daily, hourly, bedevil others; in seeking less fortunate fellow beings so that I can submerge myself in pity for the world, while congratulating my parents on their rich personal fate. When Man's Inhumanity to Man spars with my Pollyanna side, I'm flighty, moody, constantly switching loyalties.

Walking in bright, sooty sunshine, I look to justify a continuing divine irresponsibility toward ending my parents' lives. I dredge the past to recall some sufficient meanness or ugliness in them, some truly despicable trait, but can never ferret out anything authentically worthwhile. Their disagreements, their differences, their incompatibilities—whatever they may have been—were settled or suppressed in severest privacy: a pleasing legacy my husband and I have adopted, aware that our kids will probably pique their respective shrinks with the unwavering insistence that they evolve from generations of happy relationships. For years I've been embarrassed to declare—when contemporaries press for honesty—that I really like my children and my parents, and that the only man I've ever wanted to have an affair with is my husband.

*       *       *

Before his dinner every day, Mother had been feeding Dad a few teaspoonsful of fruit brandy or a soothing liqueur, which she'd bring in a small medicine bottle disguised by layers of aluminum foil. Dad has increasing difficulty now swallowing any liquid, and the mildest sweet wine is soon too strong. His poor cocktail moment has to be abandoned. Trying to sip his coffee he has a dreadful coughing spell, till the S-shaped vein in his temple turns a bright, determined blue. "No good," he rasps when the siege leaves him. "Don' wanna live."

Mother, applying the Kleenex, wiping his streaming eyes and nose, cautions: "Don't talk like that, please dear. That's not nice . . . Alicia will be here to see you on Sunday, and so will Michael, and he'll tell you all about his college. You do want to see the children, don't you?"

"Wanna be all gone . . ."

Happily there's a distraction in the hallway. Two aides are urging an old gent back to his room.

"He was climbing over the rail of the patio," one of them calls in as they pass Dad's door. "We had all we could do to pull him back off the fence."

"And you'd better watch what you're pulling there, girlie! You nearly tore my pants off . . . What is it you're getting at?" The fellow's anger mounts: "My wife tried to boss me around for sixty-eight years and I wouldn't let her. My children tried to boss me around for sixty-three years and I wouldn't let them. I'm ninety-two years old now, and I'm not going to let you boss me around either! Don't you think I'm right, sir?" he approximates a military stance, hoping to enlist Dad's support.

Right, nods Dad.

*　　*　　*

Mrs. Bellson tells me that during lunch the day before Dad had a bad experience. An olive had accidently appeared on his tray, and he'd gulped it down whole; an aide happened to be passing his room and managed to dislodge it quickly enough.

"This isn't the first time he's done something like that," she says. "Once it was a piece of meat, when the wrong tray was sent in to him; another time it was a large hard candy. I know what he has in mind . . . Sometimes I wonder if I blame him. But from now on we'll have to watch more closely—and better leave only small, easily soluble sweets around."

Later, when she brings the three o'clock body-building potion, she asks Dad, "Did you tell the folks you were weighed today?" A good prompting to activity, this: Mother and I march down the hall to the scale, then report back to Dad, comparing pounds and converting them to English stone. We ask him how much he weighs, and he replies, "Hunnert."

"How much did you say, Dad? A hundred?"

"Yeh," he answers, adding a doubtful, "Dunno." Then again, positively: "Hunnert."

This seems an exorbitant figure, since recently I'd been told in confidence that he barely pushed the indicator to eighty-six. Before we leave that day, I verify at the desk: he's lost six more pounds, but to bolster his morale, they'd told him he weighed a robust hundred.

## SEVENTEEN

"Every time I think of it, I just can't stop laughing." Mother digs into her apron pocket for a handkerchief. "Dad got such a kick out of it, he really almost laughed out loud. I haven't seen him try to laugh like that since he took sick."

Hilarity at the nursing home? Over cocktails, my husband and I yearn to hear more.

Mother explains that her brother Howard and his wife had come to lunch and then driven her over to Riverview.

"What a pair! They drive together," she tells us, "although Sybil does sit in the back seat. If you saw it in a movie, you'd say that it's silly—too much slapstick. Howard's at the wheel. He says, 'I think there's a traffic light ahead, dear. Is it green or red? I can't tell from here.' Sybil tells him it's green. He keeps going. 'No,' she yells, 'it turned red!' So he stops immediately, even though we're in the middle of the block."

Her giggle is infectious as she continues: "I tell them we have to turn at the next blinker, and Howard says, 'I know where to go, don't you worry.' Then he pokes his head way out the window and asks Sybil, 'Is it clear on the right, dear?' She tells him it's okay, so he makes a quick turn to the left. A car from the opposite direction just barely misses us. 'The hell with him,' says Howard. 'Why doesn't he look where he's going?'"

Mother is weepy with laughter, trying to subdue it.

"We go on for several blocks, and then Sybil yells, 'Howard! Be careful! Don't you see those youngsters?' A group of girls has to jump back on the sidewalk as he comes tearing along the street. 'Screwy kids,' he yells out the window. 'Wanna get your feet shortened?'

"You wouldn't believe all this could happen in such a short distance." Mother pushes up her glasses to mop at her eyes. "But that's not the end of it. We have to go round to the side street because there's no place to park in front of the building. He tries and tries to pull into a space that, I imagine, is big enough for three cars. But he can't do it—keeps bumping the curb and the fender of the car in front. 'Here, let me do it,' Sybil says. She's the impatient type, my sister-in-law is. When they change seats, I get out of the car, figuring it's a good time to leave without insulting them. So Sybil jumps into the driver's seat—she has on that charm bracelet and those little white gloves, you know—and she backs up very fast. I have to turn away, I can't watch, but Howard yells from the sidewalk, 'Stop, stop! Turn it to me—to me! There's a pole behind you!' "

Mother can hardly get the words out: " 'What pole? I don't see any pole,' Sybil yells back at him. He keeps carrying on, 'Look out—you're going to hit the pole! To me, to me, to me!' Sybil looks the other way and says, 'What are you talking about? There's no pole there.' "

Mother clutches at her sides, aching deliciously: "Of course Sybil hits the pole, but luckily there's no real damage. Then she gets out of the car, looks around very surprised, and says sheepishly, 'Gee, I really didn't see that pole.' "

Dad had been pleased to see his visitors, but Mother

couldn't wait till they left so she could share the scene with him. "Oh, Matthew, I love Howard dearly. But before I ever set foot in their car again, I'm going to take an extra one of those little white pills."

She'd repeated the story till there was no doubt Dad could visualize every detail. And till he crinkled from forehead to chin, gasping, "T'me, t'me!"

## EIGHTEEN

WE DON'T BELIEVE IT, none of us can believe it. Certainly our accountant won't believe it, Medicare notwithstanding.

Mother has to go to the hospital, jaundiced and in appalling pain. She has, it develops, a few gallstones floating around in search of a bladder. The doctor informs us that if they don't dissolve or find a compatible resting place, surgery is the only solution. However, considering the tenuous state of her health, surgery is not feasible. She may, therefore, need an operation for a condition that's inoperable.

I dread being asked, "What's new?" till I find a completely reliable answer: "Nothing much."

Mother Agatha must be at it again. Those wicked stones at last do behave, leaving Mother drained and recuperating, but reduced to a diet of nothing she enjoys. Too numerous, too extraordinary is her share of sacrifices—like forever forgoing the exotic pleasure of munching a raw carrot.

"They used to call me 'Kitten' when I was a child," she says. "Little did they know I'd have more than nine lives! How many times have I been through nonsense like this anyway?"

(That she documents attacks and operations is understandable, since they've punctuated our lives as far back as I can recall. There was once a writhing goodie, all because she'd eaten one tablespoon of ice cream—not even chocolate. I was so frightened I went from room to room, up and down the stairs, turning on all the lamps. And then back again, turning them off. In the midst of a dreadful spasm, Mother called to me as I hurried by her room, asking me to put a clean towel in the bathroom and to change the pillow cases on her bed. The doctor was coming.)

"What did you tell Dad?" a relative asks. "That Mother has a cold or something?"

"No, we told him the truth, but we did try to make it sound a little less serious."

"Surely you didn't tell him she's in the hospital?"

"Yep. We told him right away."

We amass censuring eyebrows from folks who, with misguided arrogance, often feel more competent to judge for others what they should or shouldn't know . . . the kind who lock themselves into subtle conspiracies, withholding news till they deem someone "ready to take it better." They're not unlike the little man who loved potato pancakes so much that he saved a trunkful of them in his attic.

To Mother, confined in her contacts for so long, the hospital setting is a social one once the immediate danger subsides. When an Indian intern appears, clipboard in hand, to take her medical history, she says, "You better sit down, you'll get tired standing for mine." He is thorough, however, notating data from the very beginning of her life. In answer to his first question, Mother says, "I'm never really sure how old I am because the midwife didn't report me. I'm either seventy-seven or seventy-eight. Maybe seventy-nine, but I don't think so. My mother always said, 'Thank goodness you've had your children before you're thirty.' I think I just made it."

Her birthplace? "New Jersey" is simple enough, but the three farmhouses and two barns that comprised her hometown no longer exist; neither do the records, which had burned up in an Old Courthouse fire.

And so they progress, hampered by the young doctor's difficulties with English. After taking the birthdates of her children, he asks, "Have you fiddem?"

"Beg pardon?"

"Have you fiddem?"

Mother frowns, and I'm of no help at all, though he repeats his questions several times. Finally, tapping her breast lightly with the end of his ballpoint pen, he asks, "Fid-dem?"

"Oh! Fed them! Did I breastfeed them? Oh . . . let's see . . ."

*　　*　　*

Mother quickly befriends the "sweet old lady" in the bed across the room who is constantly embarrassed by her inner gases erupting loudly, uncontrollably, in a couple of directions, often simultaneously. Mrs. Caruso laughs, just as lustily, when Mother consoles her by re-citing: "It's better to belch and bear the shame, than squelch the belch and bear the pain." We are impressed by Mrs. Caruso's exceptional sense of humor when we discover she understands only Italian. This "old lady," Mother learns, has just turned sixty-three.

*　　*　　*

Mrs. Bellson tells me that since Mother took ill, Dad has been unprecedentedly finishing everything on his breakfast and lunch trays: "Perhaps he feels he must stay healthy until she's back from the hospital."

I go to the nursing home to help him with his dinner, hoping to properly perform the established ritual. Two aides crank the bed flat, and with a "One, Two, Three," hoist Dad back onto the pillow. (This they must do several times a day, since his paralyzed parts unremittingly tug him to the foot of the bed.) Then they crank him up again and reposition him when he sags to one side. They push the tray table across his middle, and I tie his bib. Precariously upright, he unfolds his napkin and tucks it in place, straightens the paper placemat, and fingers a few spots of sloshed coffee. The tablespoon wobbles in his hand, so I offer a teaspoon—not so heavy and easier to manage.

In slow motion he sips two spoons of soup; three spoons of something brown and something green, blended separately but sharing the same bowl; three or four ounces of coffee and milk with two sugars. On the closet shelf Mother had lined up several jars of strained fruits and baby foods. There is a tin here too, with individually wrapped squares of her sponge cake. Mashed together, this is Dad's nightly dessert treat. Standing behind the tray on his "bad" side, I maneuver cup and straw; with another spoon, I catch from his chin what he can't feel when his aim is not perfect. I force myself to swallow a "That's fine!" just as Mother would say it, when he completes his measured meal.

All day I've been fanning a chill deep inside of me. By evening, knowing I'm catching cold, I breathe directly at my father, inspiring germs his way. I seek redemption through playing a tape of elevator music, and Montevanni complies by rendering "Hands Across the Table." As a frosting to my chastening process, I stop by to see Mother Agatha, who has been confounding the medics by remaining nearly hale for well over a year now.

"How is Mother feeling? And how is Dad tonight?" I audition another new fall line: "Just about the same." "That's good. God bless them." How nice one of us thinks so.

*　　*　　*

Walking back from Riverview I must set each foot only once in every box of pavement, otherwise my plan may be hexed. I shall round up all flowered plastic shopping bags in the county; I shall individually wrap in aluminum foil three dozen spoons, two dozen chocolate chip cookies, and one dozen dessert dishes with fluted rims; I shall purchase a gross of assorted Beech-Nut strained products. In the middle of the road halfway between our apartment and the convalescent home, I shall pile these items, topping them with a pair of men's size B red flannel pajama bottoms, a deck of American Airlines playing cards without the jokers, thirteen spiral-bound crossword puzzle books edited by Margaret Farrar, and the eight placemats and napkins with cross-stitched roses and back-stitch stems completed while Dad was in the hospital. At midnight on my next birthday I shall set the pile aflame, while I sit on the curb sipping from a thermos of martinis and toasting bite-size hot dog hors d'oeuvres in the bonfire.

I am about to be forty-nine years old.

*　　*　　*

At home, the Matthew Tree is doing poorly, perhaps missing Mother's steadier care. The leaves have fallen off again, this time in serious numbers, exposing a dry spray of graceful branches. As I prune half of the bush, I must pause once, abruptly, scissors in the air, unsure whether the faint whimpering, moaning, comes from within me, or from deep inside the sorry skeleton I'm dismembering.

One brittle stem, with a few flimsy leaves clinging to the top, I poke into a slim glass of water. Despite a florist's "highly unlikely" warning, I wonder if this tired sprig might take root.

# PART III

HERE WE ARE AGAIN, not much wiser, unable still to answer that explosive "Why?" I can't drag my attention back to 27 Down's four-letter Lake in Ethiopa, maybe ending in "A." Of more immediacy is arithmetic. I am absorbed in figuring precisely: Mother and I first sat in that other hospital room two thousand three hundred sixty-four days ago, plus one—or two?—for leap year. (I wonder whatever became of the teacher who enticed us with fancy math tricks, whose tour de force was proving, semiannually, that sixty-four equalled sixty-five. While he explained, the whole class believed.)

The pattern is the same, I just don't *want* to get used to it.

For once the phone call had been specific: "Your father is dying." When I reached the nursing home, Mother's face had been as white as her hair; some of the blue had washed out of her eyes. I'd seen my mother cry less than half a dozen times in the forty-odd years I've noticed her.

"Every R.N. was in here with him, five of them," she'd told me, suddenly sagging under the weight of these years. "It happened so quickly . . . Mrs. Bellson took his hand, telling him not to be afraid. And Miss Sellers just stood at the foot of the bed, crying. They're really wonderful. Dad's been like this, almost gone, since they called you." I had shaken my head, but the peculiar dizziness rocked on and on. How much longer, watching my parents watch me watch them suffer?

Next morning when they came on duty, the nurses had been a huddle of disbelief to find him there. Just barely, but there.

Dad's fever vacillates. He eats nothing for days, only some water which we drop into him occasionally through the end of a straw. At last he's conscious enough to try it for himself, but too weak to sip. An intravenous needle is pricked into his arm: "Have you ever seen anyone die of dehydration? It's awful," whispers the nurse.

How is it not awful to die? On a pointless battlefield in Vietnam? At the whim of giant avarice, or individual fury? As one of six million, martyred?

A catheter is also added to ensure against infectious "leakage." A heavy Cuban nurse appears with a bottle of irrigant swinging from an iron pole, and we leave the room while she ministers the apparatus. Later Dad rouses himself just enough to investigate the other jar on the floor under the bedrail. He traces with his eyes the course of plastic tubings, bemused at the way they're connected in and out of him. Why all this technology, employed anew to pester and prolong him?

My husband nudges me. "Poor Dad . . . all those cords . . . if they pull one, how do they know if they'll get Channel 2 or his left testicle?"

"Well, here we go again," sighs Mrs. Bellson as we pass her desk on the way home.

"Hate these long farewells . . ."

Fluent in her religion, she asks, "Don't you really think, though, in a final analysis, everyone gets his just due?"

The most devastating retort I can dream up is: "No. Do you?"

*       *       *

I bring Dad a single flower, making much of removing the printed paper and staples, the double layer of pink tissue: Any tiny, time-consuming necessity becomes a grateful activity when it can be stretched to more than fleeting interest. He opens his eyes wide. Alabaster white, each petal is carefully edged as though with a deep red magic marker. He touches the leaves, pokes at my finger lightly, wondering where the thorns are. He wriggles his chin, scrunches up his mouth, swallows a few times, closes one eye, and pleased with his accomplishment, smells it. I go down the hall to put some water in a paper container, and come back to find three aides peeking in the doorway.

"Isn't that sweet?" they whisper of Dad, who steadfastly guards the rose he clutches on his chest.

*       *       *

I am beginning to be affected:

(1) This morning I found the remains of last night's tuna fish salad in the sugar bowl's place. Happily I'd stored the sugar bowl in the refrigerator, otherwise I really would have been concerned.

(2) Out with friends the other evening, Karen'd pouted at me: "Every time we go anywhere with you people, you're always making phone calls during dinner. Is it all really *that* important?" I bid them good-bye instead of good-night.

(3) On the bus recently I'd eavesdropped over two

learned specimens discussing an article on psychology and euthanasia. "He's only working out his own death wish," they were agreeing of the author. "You don't know what the hell you're talking about," I butt in. The two professional heads had jerked upward and snug satisfaction was mine, though I did quit the bus in haste, before they could diagnose the scope of my problem or get their calling cards out of their wallets.

Those two shrinks must be specializing in ESP and sticking pins in their directories. *They* must be responsible for my Pavlovian reaction to the telephone. Every time it rings, I say to myself, sometimes out loud, "Maybe this is it." Since nothing happens when one expects it, I try *not* to anticipate my response—then perhaps the call will come. Like the kids used to say when they were very young, "You can tell me the secret now—I promise I'll forget it." I do not succeed in fooling myself into outwitting me.

The telephone, the telephone. I lean on the kitchen counter, trying to stare it into submission. I can't take a shower without hearing it, whether or not it rings. It does ring at 1 A.M.: there's no one on the line, not even a pseudo-asthmatic. It rings while I'm writing checks, listening to the Kaddish (surely a sign!) of Bloch's "Sacred Service" on WQXR: someone wants to borrow a suitcase. It rings while I'm folding laundry: my sister-in-law inquires about Dad, "I can't believe it—do you realize it's over six years?"

"I realize. Actually it's almost seven," my friendly masochism pushes for a record.

She advises me that I should be extremely proud of my father. He still can relate so well to the world. His relationship with my mother is wondrous. These years have proved the endurance—no, the transcendence—of the human spirit. "I hope he goes on forever!" she exults. We hang up. A quiver in my lower lip acts up, till I pacify it by maliciously biting all my lipstick off.

I walk through the apartment, brandishing a pair of tennis socks at every mirror, at every picture with a face in it. "She hates me! She hates me! I never knew she hated me so much!"

\* \* \*

"They painted Dad's room the other day—at least that was a little something different for him to watch." Mother is replacing the worn-out binding on a small pillow case. She'd made it a long time ago, because when she leans on Dad's bed, the blanket irritates her arms. "When they got him out of bed twice a day—at least it was something for him to look forward to. But do you realize that Dad's been in that bed, on his back, for over six months now?"

"Yes, I know. And I was there Saturday."

"Oh, that's right . . . Do you know, when the paint was dry, Dad didn't want me to put any of the pictures or cards back on the walls. He got so angry. But I insisted. Then he got involved too, and told me precisely where each one should be. I couldn't remember just where everything went . . . like those funny sketches Alicia drew of her broken toe. Dad wanted them under Richard's metal sculpture, the way they were before."

Mother pats the finished pillow, scratches a few circles around the rash on her elbow (tension-based, the doctor says), and picks up her current knitting

project: Christmas gifts for fourteen nurses. She has
seven weeks, five scarves, nine fringes to go.

❀     ❀     ❀

Only after swearing that Susan and Alicia will visit
with Dad and help him with his dinner do we persuade
Mother to attend a grandniece's wedding. She has
averaged less than one "outing" a year since Dad became ill. The kids report that they had a fine two hours,
Lish adding, "Somehow it's very secure having Pop
around, the same person, underneath, that he always
was. If we brought him an algebra problem, I bet he'd
still be able to figure it out in his head without knowing
exactly how he got the answer. It seems impossible that
a person should be able to live so long, so controlled . . .
*We* were absolutely wiped out when we left!"

They probably exhausted Dad too, but he adored
every moment of their busy program: a fashion parade
of their new clothes (including Lish's last bikini, which,
rolled up, fit into his hand); photographs of the children
in Susan's first-grade class and a booklet of pictures
they'd made for him, the top one reading, "dear pip
com hom soon i hop you are all ok." They'd braided one
another's hair by twos, threes, and fours, and badgered
him into playing a shortened version of War with the
deck of cards they'd brought.

"It's funny, the way he calls me 'Suzzy.' And he can
never manage 'Richard,' so he asked about my 'hudg-
jin.' We were so beat, we just sat down on the front steps
of the nursing home for a while after we left Pop . . . It's
dreadfully unfair for him to linger like this; but, you
know, when you're with him he's all *there* . . . "

No quarrel. My father was also there in last night's dreams.

Yes. He's there, gliding above a wide, barren plain —like the desert in *Lawrence of Arabia*—a grey, eerie light making the scene irridescent. Very soft bongo drums flutter, far away. When he realizes that I can see him, Dad floats toward me slowly, pointing his finger directly at me. I can only see his face, his arm, and that frightening finger, slowly growing larger and larger. I try to brush it away, but can't reach it. He continues steadily, bigger, closer, pointing relentlessly. First his eyes are open, fixed and haunted; but as he comes nearer they narrow to angry, then furious slits, glaring at me . . .

I was enormously relieved to wake before that finger reached me, and I lay there for a long time . . . looking at the phone . . . thinking that when Dad actually does die, it will be a great shock. Or, maybe, could he really go on forever?

It was almost daylight when I drifted back to sleep.

This time I am locked in the bathroom, spreading a few tissues on the vanitory edge. With a manicure scissors I cut open one of the sleeping pills I've been hoarding—snitching two or three from each prescription so Mother hasn't noticed. A dab from my little finger is astonishingly bitter; I eat huge gobs of mint toothpaste to wash it away. Even Dad's eroded taste-buds would balk at this sprinkled into his dessert.

Revise, revise.

Mustardy paste oozes from the inside of a vitamin.

Revise.

Tiny ferrous dots bounce gaily out into the sink, as I empty three big, ideal iron capsules, fill them instead

with the contents of ten sleeping pills, then ease together the rubbery, two-tone green coverings. I worry
that I'm not scared, not nervous. No pulse tattles anywhere, though I stop a dozen times expecting one. As I
top a small vial with cotton and stash it in the zippered
compartment of my tan leather handbag, I am thankful
for a young man recently acquitted of mercy-killing.
He'd obediently shotgunned his brother who'd pleaded
for death after being vegetablized in a motorcycle accident.

At four thirty I'm at the pet shop. At five o'clock I
am urging a new goldfish out of his temporary plastic
home and into the tank in Dad's room.

"I'd better change the filter. Should've done it last
week," I say as Mother leaves to stay overnight with my
sister. How obliging is opportunity this wintry Saturday!

"Don't forget to pull up the bedrail," Mother instructs.
"And see that there are enough tissues folded for him,
and enough mints in the tray."

"Right, right, I will."

Concerned that I'm not tense, not edgy only vaguely
impatient, I wonder, Can I do it?

"You look sleepy, Dad. I'll turn off the big light and
you can doze a while. Okay?" He murmurs appro-
priately; yes or no, I'm not sure.

Returning from the water cooler, I glance into the
dining room where two aides and a nurse are taking a
tea break.

"Active bunch of fish you've got there," one of them
calls out.

"I wish some of our patients were so well regulated,"
laughs the nurse.

"Heh heh," I agree, spreading charcoal, spun fiberglass, and paper toweling on the counter of the adjoining utility room.

In Dad's room I close the door to an inch-wide slot, opening the closet door firmly against it. Leaning sideways into the closet, I twist from his view and dump the pills from the zippered compartment of my tan leather bag to a clean handkerchief waiting in my pocket. "No germs" sounds in my head like the door-chime ad for a cosmetic canvasser. My back to the doorway, shielding us both, I offer Dad his container of water; when he opens his mouth for the straw, I slide a capsule in first. He swallows, and I ask softly, "Did that go down?" He grunts . . . Yes, I hope . . . and twice we repeat the process. He is unquestioning, incurious, nonchalantly accepting of my gift.

My hand isn't shaking, my forehead isn't damp. My heart isn't noticeably pounding. Dad reaches over and shakily helps himself to an after-dinner mint, then another. Perhaps a mite of bitterness had clung outside the seam of a capsule. He yawns, and I laugh giddily, grateful to be nervous at last.

"Sleepy? That's okay, take a nap, Dad."

I disconnect the filter and carry it to the utility room; I fuss slowly with the cleaning chore. Some fifteen minutes later Dad watches casually when I replace the rack and turn the motor on again.

"Hope I got it back right this time," I chat at the bedside, sandwiching his wisp of a hand in both of mine. His mouth opens wide, and his stiff right arm flops about accompanying the yawn. He sighs, coughs convulsively, and brings my hands toward his chin for a kiss. Then he snares another peppermint and, whirling the candy around in his mouth, settles into a babylike slumber.

"Good night, Dad, and sleep well," I recite my rote.

Above his bed the nightlight broadens his pale forehead, grooves shadows into the sunken cheeks, tugs the merest of smiles over uninhabited gums. The room is still as I tiptoe away . . .

❖   ❖   ❖

The next afternoon I am taking a roast out of the oven when the phone rings.

"I think you'd better come over." Mrs. Bellson is grave. "I've already called your sister."

Unsteadily I remove my potholder mitten, rummage for car keys, scribble a note for my husband, grab a jacket. As I'm about to slam the door behind me, I stop undecided: Did I turn off the light in the oven? I go back to check and—in deference to superstition—sit down for a moment before going out again.

Feeling foolish, then, I move slowly to the Matthew Tree slip on the window sill. The other day, routinely watering it, I'd noticed that the single sturdy white root, which had unaccountably formed, had turned a limp brown. The water had a faint odor, and those three weary leaves were tawny and shriveled. I'd washed the glass, rinsed a fuzzy film from the root, and, placing the sickly thing in fresh cool water, moved it to a sunnier spot on the sill.

Now I examine it closely. Could it be that I hadn't noticed, just beneath the water level, a minute bright green sprig popping out of the middle of the stem? Or had it pushed its way through to the light during the last several hours? I ought to rush, but I can't.

Fortunately there's little traffic. A few blocks from the nursing home, I must pull over to the side of the road. I hope I'm near the curb. I can no longer see where I'm going. I turn off the engine and sit there with the steering wheel ridging my forehead, uncontrollably sobbing.